Studying for Continuing Professional Development in Health

A guide for professionals

Kym Fraser
with **Jane Fowler, Amanda Gudmundsson, Peter Ling and Leanne Whicker**

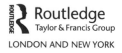
Routledge
Taylor & Francis Group

LONDON AND NEW YORK

First published 2009
by Routledge
2 Park Square, Milton Park, Abingdon, Oxon OX14 4RN

Simultaneously published in the USA and Canada
by Routledge
270 Madison Avenue, New York, NY 10016

Routledge is an imprint of the Taylor & Francis Group, an informa business

Typeset in Sabon by
GreenGate Publishing Services, Tonbridge, Kent

Printed and bound in Great Britain by
TJ International Ltd, Padstow, Cornwall

British Library Cataloguing-in-Publication Data
A catalogue record for this book is available from the British Library

Library of Congress Cataloging-in-Publication Data
Fraser, Kym, 1958–
Studying for continuing professional development in health : a guide for
professionals / Kym Fraser.
p. ; cm.
Includes bibliographical references.
1. Medicine—Study and teaching (Continuing education) I. Title.
[DNLM: 1. Health Personnel—education. 2. Learning. 3. Education,
Continuing. W 18 F841s 2009]
R845.F73 2009
610.7—dc22 2008026187

ISBN 10: 0-415-41888-7 (hbk)
ISBN 10: 0-415-41889-5 (pbk)

ISBN 13: 978-0-415-41888-1 (hbk)
ISBN 13: 978-0-415-41889-8 (pbk)

This book is dedicated to my brother Alec who is one of the brightest people I know

Contents

Figures

Tables

Author and contributors

Kym Fraser heads up the Teaching and Learning Development Group at Charles Darwin University, Australia. Kym has a career-long interest in developing effective student learning environments and has worked in this field in the UK, the USA, Australia and Hong Kong. She has worked at the University of Oxford (UK), the University of Warwick (UK), Cornell University (USA), Lingnan University (Hong Kong) and Monash University (Australia).

Kym was Director of Education for Warwick Diabetes Care in the Medical School at Warwick University from 2004 to 2007. While working at the University of Warwick, Kym and her colleagues secured over £800,000 in education development grants for their courses. The focus of their work was to develop student-centred, continuing professional development courses for health care professionals.

Kym has been an assessor for both the UK Higher Education Academy and the Australian Learning and Teaching Council. She is a past editor of the Higher Education Research and Development Society of Australasia Green and Gold Guides. Her current research interests include 'the reward and recognition of teaching', 'teaching development' and 'building teaching leadership capacity'.

Jane Fowler is a senior lecturer in the School of Human Services at Griffith University and an adjunct Professor at West Virginia University. She is convenor of the professional skills stream that is a core component of the human services programmes, incorporating courses such as Interpersonal Skills, Group Facilitation, and Counselling. Jane has extensive experience in working with and facilitating small and large groups across a range of university and private industry settings. She has developed and implemented a number of support programmes for students including 'Common Time', a practical approach to the enhancement of social and academic integration of first-year students (winner of an Australian Award for University Teaching) and the 'Tiered Mentoring Programme', which engages students with their peers and professionals. Jane has developed a wide range of materials and resources for interpersonal and group work.

Amanda Gudmundsson is a senior lecturer in the School of Management at Queensland University of Technology. She teaches in the fields of human resource management and professional skills development. Amanda has gained substantial experience facilitating groups through the incorporation of group-based approaches to learning in her teaching. Through her teaching and research activities Amanda has developed an appreciation of the issues and concerns experienced by students participating in group-based learning.

Peter Ling is Associate Dean, Swinburne Professional Learning, Swinburne University of Technology, Melbourne. Peter has extensive experience in educational development at RMIT University and Swinburne University of Technology. He was principle researcher in several national projects including The Development of Academics and Higher Education Futures (Carrick Institute of Learning and Teaching in Higher Education, 2008) and The Effectiveness of Models of Flexible Provision of Higher Education in Australia (Department of Education Training and Youth Affairs, 2001). Peter was co-researcher for Multiple Modes of Delivery, A Higher Education Innovation Program project of the Australian Universities Teaching Committee, 2004, and *New Directions in Resource Based Learning: Quality, Equity and Costs*, report to the Higher Education Council, Canberra, 1997. Peter authored 'From a community of scholars to a company' in K. Fraser (ed.) *Education Development and Leadership in Higher Education: Developing an Effective Institutional Strategy*, London, RoutledgeFalmer, 2005, and co-authored with A. Inglis and V. Joosten *Delivering Digitally: Managing the Transition to the Knowledge Media*, London, Kogan Page, 1999.

Leanne Whicker has a background in organisational development consulting and human resources management. In her early career, she provided consulting services for a range of clients in the agricultural, health foods, mining, and metal industries. More recently Leanne has held senior human resource management roles in the financial services sector, and has worked as an internal consultant for a large energy distributor in Queensland, leading cultural change. Throughout her career to date, Leanne has worked closely with project teams, management teams, temporary work groups and student groups to facilitate their interactions and develop their potential to perform effectively. Much of this work has drawn on her qualifications and experience as an organisational psychologist to work with both individual team members' needs and group needs, within the dynamics and constraints of the team task and process. Leanne has a special interest in group facilitation, organisational development and change, knowledge management and human resources management. Leanne has lectured at Griffith University and Queensland University of Technology.

Preface

I have been interested in student learning for as long as I can remember. As an undergraduate it puzzled me that some of my friends, no matter how hard they studied, still failed or only just passed their subjects. I had always held the belief that if a person studied 'hard' enough, any subject was understandable. As a young secondary school science/maths teacher it became apparent to me that studying 'hard' or 'harder' wasn't necessarily enough for all students to pass or do well. Students needed to know 'how to learn'. There are many different ways of learning and as students we need to be able to choose the ways in which we learn.

My career progressed and I moved into the university sector where I undertook a PhD. Through my studies and work I learnt a great deal about the different ways in which students learn and the different ways in which teachers can develop useful student learning environments.

The genesis of this book came about through my role with Warwick Diabetes Care at the University of Warwick where I and my colleagues worked to provide excellent learning opportunities for health care professionals seeking to undertake university study as part of their continuing professional development. For many of our students it had been a long time since they had studied at university and some of our students hadn't studied at university before. This book is written for all health care students: the experienced and the inexperienced, those with degrees and those without, those studying undergraduate courses and those studying postgraduate courses. I hope that you both enjoy and find value in reading this book and that it helps you to think about how you learn, and most importantly, how your learning can influence your health care practice.

Acknowledgements

I have been fortunate in my career to have had many colleagues from whom and with whom I have learnt a great deal about our profession and our discipline. 'Collegial' is the overwhelming sense that I have of these individuals and I am grateful for their friendship and their willingness to share their insights and understanding with me.

My thanks to Grace McInnes and Eloise Cook for their efforts in bringing this book to publication.

Alec, I have known and loved you for all of my life. You always had faith in me and for your faith, friendship and support, I am truly grateful. This book is dedicated to you.

My heartfelt thanks and more to Susie for your unfailing moral and intellectual support, your kindness and good humour, the reassuring 4a.m. conversations, the everyday things that you took on so I could 'work on the book' and the not so everyday things; like your willingness to move country with me.

My mother left school in 1936 at the age of sixteen. In spite of not having a tertiary education she always maintained that 'an education was no load to carry'. Her encouragement and support underpinned my academic achievements and I am indebted to her in so very many ways.

Special thanks to my colleagues in both Australia and the UK who reviewed the chapters of this book; Sue Rivers, Anne McDermott, Sue Hamilton, Sandra Dunn, Sharon Watson and Marguerite Maher.

Many thanks to my Charles Darwin University colleagues Paula Wilson and Elisabet Reiten-Griffith for producing the concept maps in this book, Antonio Senga for helping me with the style template and Amander Dimmock for illustrating Figures 2.1, 3.2 and 3.3.

In particular I would like to thank my chapter contributors, Peter Ling, Jane Fowler, Amanda Gudmundsson and Leanne Whicker for their excellent work.

I am indebted to Anne McDermott (2004–7 Course Director for the Warwick Diabetes Care Certificate in Diabetes Care, University of Warwick) who gave me permission to use the criteria and guidelines that Warwick Diabetes Care developed for the student research assignment used in its certificate. I have modified the criteria and guidelines for the purposes of this book.

I wish to thank Professor Sandra Dunn of Charles Darwin University for allowing me to use the grading system guidelines that the School of Graduate Health Practice uses in its assessment of written work. I have slightly modified the guidelines for the purposes of this book.

My thanks to Australian Academic Press for allowing Jane Fowler, Amanda Gudmundsson and Leanne Whicker permission to reproduce excerpts from their book *Groups Work* (2006).

Finally my thanks to the Higher Education Research Society of Australasia for giving me permission to reproduce excerpts from the Green Guide that I wrote for the society, *Student Centred Teaching: The Development and Use of Conceptual Frameworks* (1996).

Introduction

This book is written for health care professionals (HCPs). It's written for HCPs who are contemplating returning to study after many years and it's written for those who are currently enrolled in their degree, graduate certificate, graduate diploma or similar. Over the years that I have worked in universities, the focus of my work has been the improvement of student learning. Through teaching and working with many academics during my career, I have learnt a lot about how students learn, what university level study requires and the sorts of barriers that prevent students, especially mature age students, from achieving success in their studies.

As an undergraduate I knew a mature age student who studied incredibly hard and yet always struggled to pass her subjects and often failed them. Many years later, I came to understand the ways in which she probably could have been helped to 'learn how to learn' (Novak and Gowin, 1984). Working 'harder' by spending more time learning in the same ways doesn't always lead to academic success. Students often need to learn differently and this book helps students and prospective students to understand the many different ways there are to learn.

The book is structured to guide the reader through the preparatory stages for study: choosing the course[1] of study, discussing study time needs with family and friends, and setting up for and managing study (Chapters 1 and 2). Then we discuss what learning is and the different ways that students can learn and the strategies that teachers use to help students to learn (Chapters 3 and 4). The book next explores two of the most common ways in which students are assessed: written assignments and exams (Chapters 5 and 6). The book finishes with a discussion of the ways in which students may need to work: online and in groups (Chapters 7 and 8). The reader may choose to read the book from beginning to end or to read specific chapters or parts of chapters, depending upon individual need.

In the following chapters I discuss in detail the preparation, approaches, strategies and different ways of learning that students can use in their study. Each chapter begins with an example of learning outcomes which indicates some of the things that students can expect to be able to do or know having read the chapter. The learning outcomes aren't an exhaustive list. Each chapter also ends with a paragraph describing the next chapter. Several chapters have a 'Tips' section at the end of the chapter which highlights other useful ideas on the topic. Many chapters include websites that can be accessed to explore the chapter topics further. Here I provide a brief overview of each of the chapters to give readers a sense of what each chapter discusses.

Chapter 1, 'Preparing to study', explores the different types of continuing professional development (CPD) that are available and strategies to help you choose the type of CPD most useful to your needs. The chapter also identifies questions to ask a course teacher before enrolling in a course.

Chapter 2, 'Study management', discusses the nitty gritty of managing your study, such as where to keep your notes, planning a study timetable, talking with family about the time you need to study and the support you need from them to do the course. The chapter also encourages you to talk with relevant support staff for your course, such as librarians and the disability officer if you have a disability.

Chapter 3, 'Learning', identifies different ways to learn and provides ideas about how students can take advantage of the ways in which teachers structure their teaching to help students to learn. The chapter talks about the need for students to be strategic about how they learn as there is always a lot to do when studying and some ways of learning are more time intensive than others. Students can choose how they will spend their study time.

Chapter 4, 'Concept mapping: a strategy to make meaning', demonstrates one technique that can be used to help students to make sense of their study and also help students to take concise notes. The technique of concept mapping helps students to articulate how concepts are related to each other. Linking concepts in this way helps students to learn about the concepts. The technique is one that can be learnt quickly and can be used to develop an outline for an assignment or produce easy-to-read summaries for exam preparation.

Chapter 5, 'Writing', is the longest chapter in the book. We write in our everyday lives and many of the things that we do when we write are the things that we need to do in our academic writing. There are also other things to know about academic writing and once we know those things we can make improvements. Among other things this chapter discusses the planning of a writing timetable, one approach to writing an assignment, addressing the marking criteria for an assignment and the structure of three different assignment types.

Chapter 6, 'Preparing for and taking exams', discusses the different strategies we can use to prepare for an exam, and the choices to be made about how prepared to be. It isn't always possible to be 100 per cent prepared for an exam and there are choices that we can make about the level of our preparation. The chapter also discusses specific strategies that can be used in the exam to try to maximise marks.

Chapter 7, 'Learning online', discusses the responsibilities of studying online and the strategies that can be used to study successfully. Associate Professor Peter Ling from Swinburne University of Technology has written a very pragmatic chapter which will be relevant for students who have never studied online before as well as for students who want to improve their online learning experiences.

Chapter 8, 'Working in groups', is written by the authors Dr Jane Fowler (Griffith University), Dr Amanda Gudmundsson (Queensland University of Technology) and Dr Leanne Whicker, who wrote the very successful guide *Groups Work* (2006). Health care professionals work in teams in their everyday work and the usefulness of the ideas and strategies discussed in the group work chapter will extend well beyond your student days and into your career as a health care professional.

Learning is something that we do every day and it can be a real pleasure. I wish you every success with your future studies and I hope that you find the ideas in this book useful.

1   Preparing to study

Learning outcomes

By the end of this chapter readers are expected to be able to:

- identify different types of continuing professional development (CPD)
- articulate reasons for choosing a particular type of CPD, and
- identify questions to ask a course teacher before enrolling in a course.

Introduction

Health care professionals (HCPs) engage in continuing professional development (CPD) as a matter of course throughout their careers. On a day-to-day basis CPD can be as informal as learning on the job by watching colleagues or reading professional journals and magazines. Regularly the CPD in which we engage is more formal; for example supervision of our work by a colleague, attending workshops and enrolling in accredited courses. While formal CPD is the focus of this book, the ideas of learning that we discuss can equally be applied to the informal CPD in which we regularly engage.

Enrolling in an accredited course, regardless of the level or length of commitment that is required, can be daunting. Any course that we take will require a commitment, not just from us but often from our families and our employers. In this chapter I want to discuss that commitment in terms of the reasons for enrolling in a course, impact on family, and the impact on us as individuals.

Preparing to undertake formal CPD

When it comes to learning, we have choices and it really helps to know what those choices are so we can make conscious decisions about how we plan to engage with CPD. Believe it or not, the reasons why we undertake formal CPD can influence the ways in which we choose to engage with the course; they can influence the ways in which we choose to learn. Reasons for engaging in CPD include:

- we need a particular qualification to remain in our current position or to move into another position
- we want to learn new skills in order to improve our practice
- we want to improve our understanding in order to improve our practice, and
- our employer wants us to enrol in a specific CPD course.

This isn't an exhaustive list and it is highly likely that more than one reason underpins our choosing to study. Put simply, if we enrol in a course because we need the qualification, and we aren't particularly concerned with what we learn from the course, we may choose to put in a minimum effort just to pass the course. We can choose to memorise information, knowing that while this is quicker than learning for understanding, it is unlikely that we will remember this information much past the assessment of the course. On the other hand, if we want to enhance our understanding and learn new skills, then we will need to study in such a way that we can make sense of the course, for example by applying new ideas to our work environment, choosing our assignment topics so that they can influence the work that we do, and so on. Different ways of learning is the topic of Chapter 3. There is nothing wrong with being strategic about how you choose to study. What's important is that you know that there are different ways to learn and that there are pros and cons with each way.

Choosing the course that is right for you

So what sort of CPD makes sense for you at this time in your life? The reasons why we want to undertake CPD will help us to choose the CPD opportunity that will be of most use to us. Table 1.1 shows a range of possibilities, from enrolling in a master's level course through to having a company representative demonstrate a new product. If it makes sense for you to take a course, and you have determined the level (non-accredited/accredited/postgraduate/undergraduate level), you may find that there are numerous options from which you can choose. Your time is precious and it is important to check out the alternatives so that you choose the course that is most relevant and useful to you. There are some common factors to look for in a course, regardless of the level of course. Are there clear opportunities for you to seek the support of teachers? Will the assessment help you to learn and to apply information to your work context? Is there a mix of learning opportunities provided (e.g. group work, case studies, lectures, etc.)? It is worth investigating a couple of courses to determine which one suits you best. Course descriptions and frequently asked questions (FAQs) are usually provided on the institution's website.

Table 1.1 Different reasons for undertaking continual professional development (CPD) can influence the type of CPD that may be relevant

Reason for undertaking CPD	Type of CPD that may be appropriate
Promotion requires a particular qualification – e.g. a master's degree.	University-accredited courses or courses from the relevant professional body. Talk with colleagues about their experiences of courses available and select one that suits your requirements.
Need to learn a discrete skill, or a discrete set of information – e.g. about a new drug.	A practical workshop; a meeting with a company representative; one-to-one demonstration from a peer; supervision etc.
Need to understand a substantial area of information and skills and demonstrate that you have that understanding.	Assessed undergraduate or postgraduate level, accredited course or module; a series of interrelated workshops; professional journal articles or books combined with supervision.
Requirement for your practice, such as a Nursing and Midwifery Council requirement.	Accredited course.

Advice from colleagues can be invaluable. In particular, colleagues who have taken a course in which you are considering enrolling can comment knowledgeably on the course and the teaching of the course (refer to the section 'Ways teachers help students to learn' in Chapter 3 to see the sorts of things that constitute good teaching practice). I also suggest taking the time to talk with the course director or teacher. Talk with them about any aspects that you want insight into. Find out what their role is and what support they can provide you with to help you to complete the course successfully. You may want to find out how much study time you will need each week, what resources are provided, what the assessments are and what equipment you might need (for example a computer with internet access). You might also ask to be put in touch with a recent student of the course. It will be your precious time and effort that you spend on the course. A little 'homework' in choosing the right course can make the world of difference to your learning experience.

Time commitment and support

Completing a CPD course takes time and effort. Even if our employer provides time to attend the workshop/course, we will need to devote our own time to complete the assessments and study requirements. Doing so is often at the cost of spending time with family and friends or pursuing other activities. It's highly likely that your own time already has many demands placed upon it. For example, you may have family responsibilities such as shopping for an elderly parent, your share of household responsibilities (cooking/cleaning/grocery shopping/bill paying and so on), child care, etc.

To enrol in a course of study, you will need periods of uninterrupted time when you feel able to study and you may well need to negotiate support to make this time available. (This aspect is discussed further in Chapter 2.)

Having chosen to do a course that will require commitment of your own time outside of work, it's important to involve the people in your life if you anticipate needing their support and understanding. Do the people in your life who can support you:

- know why you are taking the course?
- understand how much time you will need each week to devote to this work?, and
- know what you need from them in order for you to succeed?

Before undertaking a course it is useful to articulate the reasons for studying, the barriers to studying and ways to engage family and friends in helping you to successfully complete the course.

Ourselves as learners

Confidence and motivation are keys to learning, as they are to most things in life. Sometimes our confidence about learning is low because of our learning experiences earlier in life. We need to remember that we learn all of the time in our everyday lives. We learnt to drive (perhaps), we learn to use new systems and processes at work, many of us learnt how to raise children, etc. The list is endless. Every one of us knows how to learn in particular situations and every one of us can learn how to learn for formal CPD. Like most things, becoming better at learning takes some practice, time and thought.

It takes time to develop all of the elements that contribute to the successful completion of CPD courses (e.g. writing, reading, study strategies, learning approaches). Be kind to yourself. Your work will improve with time, effort, feedback and reflection. Only you can give yourself the opportunity to improve. Sometimes you will need a tip or a strategy to improve; at other times you will need something more substantive than a 'quick fix'. You may need to rethink your approaches and experiment to find what works best for you. This book will help you to think about and practise your learning. Your family, friends and colleagues may also be helpful. We will explore 'learning' in Chapter 3.

Case studies

In this book you will be introduced to three different fictional health care professionals or 'characters'. In many of the chapters a character's particular situation, struggles and successes will be explored in relation to the topic of the chapter. The characters are representative of different types of real-life situations. One of the characters may reflect your situation or perhaps particular issues and concerns that are relevant to you may be found in different characters. My reason for including each of these characters is to make the ideas found in the chapters come alive and make sense.

Marisa

Marisa is a forty-three-year-old registered nurse who has recently taken up a position as a practice nurse in a local GP clinic. The clinic has six full-time doctors, two practice nurses, a health care support worker and two receptionists. The practice has decided to run a monthly diabetes clinic and Marisa has been asked to run the clinic. Marisa has never run a diabetes clinic and knows very little about diabetes.

Marisa and Susan, one of the practice GPs, have discussed the professional development and support that Marisa will need to help her to take on this responsibility. There are lots of different possibilities from which to choose. There are several one-day diabetes workshops that Marisa can attend, or she can read a diabetes text or journal articles, or she can enrol in a university-accredited course at the graduate or undergraduate level. Because of the knowledge and skill level required, they have agreed that Marisa will enrol in an undergraduate level course of 20–30 credit points. Susan has agreed that the clinic will pay for the course and provide Marisa with time to attend any face-to-face commitments. Marisa will study and write assignments in her own time. Also, Marisa will observe several clinics of the diabetes specialist nurse (DSN) in the local diabetes team and will be supervised by the DSN for the first three months of clinics that Marisa holds. After that she will call the local diabetes team if she needs advice or is uncertain about the care of a diabetes patient.

Ben

Ben is twenty-two and has worked in various jobs since finishing his A levels when he was eighteen. After spending two months in hospital as a patient he decided that he wants to work as a health care professional. He has been accepted to do a Diploma of General Nursing at the local university. Ben is about to start his first year of the course and has moved into his parents' home.

Kris

Kris is fifty-one years old and is a ward sister of a twenty-four-bed surgical ward. She is responsible for managing a junior ward sister, six staff nurses and eight health care support workers. Kris works 9a.m–5p.m. in her current role. She did her training in her late thirties and became a nurse at forty when her children were teenagers. Kris is a single parent.

She has been a ward sister for two years and is interested in applying for promotion to manager of the surgical ward. This role would increase her responsibilities to include budget holding, development of protocols, staff CPD, and development of the service, and increase the number of wards within her remit. In her recent appraisal Kris and her line manager agreed that Kris would do the Diploma in Health Service Management through the Royal College of Nursing Institute. To do this course Kris will need to complete six, undergraduate level-2, 20-credit-point modules. They are each fourteen weeks long and Kris expects to complete the course within two years.

The next chapter

In this chapter we discussed choosing the course that will meet your learning needs, engendering support from family and friends to help you complete your course of study and we briefly touched on building confidence to study. In the next chapter we will look at the nitty gritty specifics of managing our study – where and when to study, motivation to study, planning our study and studying with people.

2   Study management

> **Learning outcomes**
>
> By the end of this chapter readers are expected to be able to:
>
> - choose an appropriate place to study
> - plan a weekly study schedule, trial it and change it if necessary
> - develop a study plan for the length of the course
> - experiment with note taking, and
> - identify which resources they will explore (library, disability office, etc.).

Introduction

When we return to study, there are some basic skills that can greatly assist us to complete a course successfully. Teachers often assume that students have these skills and understandably do not devote precious course time to discussing them. However, it is precisely a lack of understanding of these skills that can influence a student's ability to complete a course successfully. In this chapter we will discuss: where to study, when to study, keeping motivated, making and experimenting with study plans, taking notes and reflecting and improving.

Place of study

While you may find that you do some of your study on the train or you do some reading on the couch or in bed, having a specific place to study is incredibly useful. Psychologically, your study space is for studying and completing assessments. If you study in a space that is also used for other activities, you may find that during your study time you get involved in non-study activities associated with that space; for example if you study at the kitchen table, you may find yourself washing up during your study time.

You can use your study space to store and file your notes and books so that everything you need is in the one place and to hand. It may help your family not to disturb you when they also associate your need for uninterrupted time with your being in a particular space. A study place does not always need to be at home. You may choose to keep all of your study needs together in one place, such as a book bag, and go to your work place, a friend's home or the local library to study.

Wherever you have your study place, you will need good light, a comfortable chair, comfortable temperature, a desk and in all likelihood a computer. It is important for you to make sure that your desk set-up provides you with a good posture so that you don't have a sore neck and shoulders from reading and working on the computer. A search of the web will provide you with information on ergonomics, for example, Ergonomics in Australia: http://www.ergonomics.com.au/. You will also need pens and pencils, paper, folders, a stapler, a good dictionary (perhaps on your computer), a clock and possibly a hole punch. Different courses will have different requirements and some courses may require you to have a calculator, graph paper, internet access and equipment to play a DVD.

Keep all of your written materials together (e.g. your notes, course handbook, handouts, copies of articles). File them as you get them. It may make sense to have a separate folder for copies of articles and printouts from websites that you collect, or it might make more sense to put particular copies with particular topic areas that you are studying. What's important is that you systematically organise all of the materials for your course, whether that's in loose-leaf folders or hanging files or notebooks. It can be a tremendous waste of time to have to search the house/car/office for that one article that you found in the library a month ago.

Motivation and procrastination

When we first start a course our motivation levels are often high. It's not unusual though for our motivation level to drop at times during the course. There can be lots of reasons for a drop in motivation. Dawson (2004) suggests that before starting a course it can be useful to write down the reasons for doing the course and then keep that list of reasons. When you feel dispirited, rereading the list and revisiting those reasons may lift your spirits.

Even if our motivation to enrol in a course comes from an external source (e.g. necessary for promotion, a career change, etc.), our motivation for sticking with the course day in and day out will come from ourselves. Procrastination is a problem with which many of us struggle. It's the starting that is often the problem. Once we start our study for the day, we often find that we can 'stick with it'.

> Studying sometimes produces a sense of drifting in a sea of meaninglessness. This leads you to clutch at any straws of distractions that you

can find. When you don't really understand the text or you don't really know what you are trying to achieve, you feel restless and uneasy.

Distractions offer you a chance to focus your attentions on familiar and meaningful parts of your life and so escape from the uncertainties of studying. Our urge to avoid uncertainty is very strong. That is why it is so important to define tasks for yourself to create a pattern and a meaning to your work.

(Northedge *et al.*, 1997, p. 11)

So, let's talk about 'uncertainty' and 'starting'. What's the problem with 'uncertainty' and 'starting'? Often we lack confidence that we can do whatever it is that we need to do. There's so much to do and the whole lot is daunting. One strategy to help reduce the uncertainty and to help us start our work is to break down what we need to do into little pieces that seem 'doable'. 'I'll just read the first two pages of the next chapter and see how that goes.' You don't even have to take notes – just read the first few pages and then see how you are feeling. (Please note that it is important that you are actually studying and not doing something like tidying your desk, which is study management.) Break down the work into small pieces and work through them one piece at a time. The Chinese proverb that a journey of a thousand miles must begin with a single step applies to our own study.

The other element that influences our motivation to study is that we tend to be very good at being critical of ourselves. Self-belief and feeling successful are important parts of motivating yourself to continue with your course. Celebrate the little successes as you go; it's great that you read that chapter during your study time today – well done you. Recognise where you are successful and give yourself permission to feel good about those successes.

As you begin and continue your study you will identify strategies that help you to stick with your study during your study time. For example, it may not be useful to assume that initially you will be able to sit down and fully concentrate on your study for an entire hour. You may need to build up to studying for an hour. Perhaps initially you can concentrate on your work for fifteen-minute slots, with three- or four-minute 'stretch or make a cup of coffee or walk into the garden to smell the flowers' breaks in between. At the end of an hour you might choose to give yourself a fifteen-minute break before starting again. You might find it easier to stick with your study if you mix up your study tasks in each session. For example, read one chapter, look online for a reference on a particular topic, summarise your notes from the tutorial. Whatever you do, use your time to good effect. Ineffective use of study time is a waste of your time and will probably leave you feeling guilty. You may as well do something else that you want or need to do rather than just fill in your study time in an ineffective way.

One of the key concepts that we have been talking about in this section on motivation and procrastination is time management. All throughout our lives we manage our time, whether it's with respect to work, household work, hobbies, or time with family and friends. When it comes to our study we also need to manage our time and use it effectively. For many of us time is a very precious resource and we don't want to waste it. There are many websites that discuss further issues of time management. Here are two that you may find of use: 'Time management tips from students' – Middlesex University: http://www.mdx.ac.uk/www/study/Timetips.htm and 'Managing time' – Study Guides and Strategies: http://www.studygs.net/timman.htm.

When to study

There are a number of elements that influence when it is best for an individual to study. There will be times during a twenty-four-hour period when you are more alert and better able to do the academic work required for your course. Some people rise early in order to have uninterrupted time before the rest of the family get up. They are probably 'early morning' people who function well at that time. Others find that they work best later in the evenings, and this may fit well with family responsibilities. Still others may find dedicating time during the weekends to be best for them. Some people work part-time or shift work and are able to dedicate a section of a week-day as their study time.

To determine when you might best study you will need to know 1) what your week typically looks like, and 2) how much time you need each week for study. Then, knowing when in the day you are most alert, make a plan for your study. It's useful to have chunks of time for study; at least an hour at any one time. Try making a schedule of your week like Marisa's schedule shown in Table 2.1.

Marisa

Table 2.1 Marisa's weekly schedule

Time	Monday	Tuesday	Wednesday	Thursday	Friday	Saturday	Sunday
Morning	Children to school Go to work	Children to school Go to work	Children to school Go to work	Children to school Go to work	Children to school Go to work	Study 8– 12.30	Washing and house-work
After-noon	Work	Work	Work	Work	Work	Children's football match	To Mum and Dad for lunch
Evening	Children to football classes	House-work and bills	Study 5.15– 6.45 7 collect children	Washing and weekly shopping			

Marisa is the practice nurse who is taking charge of her practice's monthly diabetes clinic. Marisa has enrolled in an accredited 30-credit-point, undergraduate diabetes course. The course runs over nine months, has six face-to-face meetings and several assessment elements. Marisa has three teenage children and a partner who regularly travels away from home for work during the week. Marisa's attitude towards her work has really improved since taking up her new diabetes role and her partner is keen for her to continue to be happy in her work. Marisa has talked with the course director who suggested that over the nine months of the course, she would need to commit approximately five hours a week for study, homework and assessment. Marisa and her partner have agreed that as she is often the only parent at home during the week, the best time for Marisa to study is at the weekends. Marisa's partner will look after the children and household responsibilities every Saturday until 1p.m. Marisa is an early morning person so she plans to start her study by 8a.m. With three teenagers in the house she has decided not to try to study at home. She has arranged access to her workplace so that she can study at work and has one shelf on the bookshelf cleared for all of her study materials. Also on a Wednesday afternoon the three children have football practice and she doesn't have to pick them up until 7p.m. Marisa plans on spending one to one-and-a-half hours after work studying on Wednesday afternoons.

Sticking to a schedule can be hard. In the first week you may manage only half of the study time that you planned. Try to be positive; you have made a start on your study and next week you will do a little more than you did this week. Try out your schedule for a couple of weeks. After this trial, think about whether the plan is working for you or if you would be best to reorganise your study schedule. Don't simply stick with a schedule that isn't working. You are the person responsible for coming up with a schedule that works for you so be prepared to experiment with your time and your timing.

Ben

Ben is taking a full-time course. Sixty per cent of the week is spent in classes and forty per cent is spent in clinical practice settings. On top of those face-to-face commitments, the course requires students to spend twenty hours a week in study time. Ben hasn't studied for four years and in his first week he found it difficult to sit down for three hours at a stretch and concentrate on his work. His girlfriend Anne suggested that initially he breaks the three-hour session up into half-hour chunks. At the end of half an hour he could reward himself with a five- to ten-minute break. He could go to the kitchen and eat a sweet treat, make a cup of coffee, do some stretching exercises. The downside was that this added an extra half an hour or more to his study sessions; however, each week Ben gradually increased the time until he was working for an hour at a time.

Table 2.2 Ben's weekly schedule

Time	Monday	Tuesday	Wednesday	Thursday	Friday	Saturday	Sunday
Morning	Classes	Classes	Classes	Classes	Classes		
Afternoon	Hospital	Hospital	Hospital	Hospital	Study 3 hours	Study 4 hours	Study 4 hours
Evening	Study 3 hours		Study 3 hours	Study 3 hours			

After three weeks Ben decided that his plan to work in the mornings before classes wasn't working. He usually stayed at Anne's place on a Friday evening and didn't want to change that. He and Anne agreed that he would leave her place by 11a.m. at the weekends so that he could study in the afternoons and still go out on Friday and Saturday evenings (Table 2.2). It will take considerable resolve for both Ben and Anne to ensure that this new schedule works.

You may also wish to experiment with what you do when. Some things you can do in short periods of time or when you are tired (e.g. organise notes, plan what you need to look for in the library, find and bookmark websites). Other things will need a longer period of time when you feel alert (e.g. reading a chapter and taking notes, writing the introduction to your assignment). How you use a block of time might need to be carefully considered. For instance, if you have a three-hour study block, you might be best to spend the first hour reading materials that are 'dense' when your concentration is at its best. Later in the study block you can summarise your notes from a class, look on the web for information, and contribute to the online discussion.

If you are going to study, it's likely that your study will need to be prioritised above some other things in your life. It's important to recognise that making the time to study may require a sacrifice of some sort. Try not to feel guilty about putting your studies before your family sometimes. You may need to negotiate some ground rules with your family so that you can have enough quiet time to study, free from distraction.

Planning your study

There are different elements to planning your study and in this chapter we will look at two key elements: fitting your studying into the length of the course and setting yourself specific tasks to do each week.

Timelines

Timelines help to bring structure and strategy to study. We can use timelines to break the time of the course up into manageable chunks that we can work towards achieving every time we sit down to study. Timelines also help us to meet assignment and exam deadlines. At the beginning of the course, it is very useful to create your timeline of due dates and then work backwards from there to determine when you need to start work on specific assessments.

Kris

Kris's first module is taught over fourteen weeks. During those fourteen weeks five topics will be taught and each topic takes two to three weeks to cover. The module has an end-of-module exam in week 14 and a project which is to be completed within two months of the end of the fourteenth week. The teacher has provided students with two past papers for exam practice. Kris has made a study plan to help her to improve her chances of doing well in the exam (Table 2.3). She has decided that she would like to do the first practice exam at the beginning of week 12 even though she won't have finished topic 5. She wants to do the first practice exam then so that she will have time to revise any areas that the practice exam highlights that she doesn't understand. She would then expect to take the second practice exam on the weekend at the beginning of week 14.

Kris believes that to make best use of the practice exams, she will need to have studied the topic areas beforehand. Please note that the plan in Table 2.3 has yet to contain anything about reading in preparation for each topic or writing the project that is also part of the assessment. We will discuss these aspects more fully in later chapters. This table illustrates how to work backwards from a 'due date' so you can plan your exam study time effectively.

Table 2.3 Exam study plan

Weeks	Topic	Study
Week 1	1	
Week 2	1	
Week 3	2	Revise topic 1 and summarise
Week 4	2	
Week 5	2	
Week 6	3	Revise topic 2 and summarise
Week 7	3	Read topic 1 summary
Week 8	3	
Week 9	4	Revise topic 3 and summarise
Week 10	4	Read topic 2 summary
Week 11	4	Read topic 3 summary
Week 12	5	Revise topic 4 and summarise, do practice exam 1
Week 13	5	Look up topic areas highlighted as needing more work in practice exam 1
Week 14	Exam	Revise topic 5 and summarise, do practice exam 2

Specifying study tasks

Each week you need to know what you need/want to achieve in the week. Try ending every week of study by making your list of what to do in the following week. Your list might include reading and summarising so many pages or chapters of a textbook, going to the library to search for and copy or make notes from certain references, talking with a colleague about a particular national guideline, writing so many words for an assignment, etc. Setting yourself specific chunks of work that you can do in the week will help you to get started and to keep working. It's both satisfying and motivating to know that you have finished what you set yourself to do.

Setting work takes practice. At first you may set yourself too much or too little. In time you will come to know just how long different things take you to do and this will help you to set realistic tasks to do in the time that you have. Try not to be discouraged. You actually aren't the slowest reader in the world or incapable of writing a sentence. Reading chapters, finding references, etc. all take time and sometimes a lot longer than we would have credited.

Feeling behind in your work seems to be the lot of being a student. It is not unusual to feel behind from the very first day of a course. It may not be humanly possible to do all of the suggested pre-reading. As students we need to be strategic in how we use our study time. So, you might choose to read only the required textbook (if one has been listed) and not any of the fifteen recommended references. Or you might choose to read the text and three of the references, or parts of five of the references. You can always talk with your teacher about how to select what to read from the references. All of these strategic decisions will depend upon: your own available time; what you will need to do to pass the course; and what you want to get out of the course (a pass, complete understanding, etc.). Try to keep your spirits up and to keep going with your study. Keeping in contact with someone else doing the course may help you both with your motivation.

Taking notes

There is every chance that in your course you will read a lot over many months. Information that you read last week let alone three months ago is likely to disappear from your memory. Reading with the purpose of taking notes helps you to:

- focus your attention as you read
- make sense of what you are reading, and
- develop a summary of your reading that you can access more easily than returning to the original text/article/website.

Your notes are written for you, not for anyone else. They have to make sense to you and you alone. When reading we need to ask ourselves at least three key questions:

1   Do I need to take notes from this reading?
2   If so, what level of detail do I need in my notes?
3   What do I need to understand from my reading?

We probably won't have the time to take detailed notes of all of the things that we read. So we need to be strategic and selective. One thing to avoid is simply copying what we read into our notes. What we need to do when taking notes is pull out the main ideas and capture them in a way that makes sense to us. We have to read the materials and make sense of them. The author of what you are reading has made an argument or explained a set of ideas and when you have understood the explanation/argument, your notes need to reflect what you have understood to be the key ideas and how those ideas are linked together.

If you haven't taken notes for a long time or you aren't confident about your note taking, just have a go. It doesn't matter initially how you write your notes, so long as you have written something. Then you can improve your technique. I suggest that you take your notes of an article or chapter and talk with your teacher about these notes (or a colleague or another student taking the course). Do your notes capture the key ideas of the reading? Are they structured in a useful way? Are they too dense/sparse? How could you improve your notes? These are all useful questions to discuss with others and having a specific example of your notes will help the discussion proceed.

Below is a paragraph from *Lewis's Medical–Surgical Nursing* (Brown and Edwards, 2005), a common nursing degree text used in Australia. After the quoted paragraph are three sets of notes from the paragraph showing different levels of detail.

STRUCTURES AND FUNCTIONS OF THE RESPIRATORY SYSTEM
The primary purpose of the respiratory system is gas exchange, which involves the transfer of oxygen and carbon dioxide between the atmosphere and the blood. The respiratory system is divided into two parts: the upper respiratory tract and the lower respiratory tract … The upper respiratory tract includes the nose, pharynx, adenoids, tonsils, epiglottis, larynx and trachea. The lower respiratory tract consists of the bronchi, bronchioles, alveolar ducts and alveoli. With the exception of the right and left mainstem bronchi, all lower airway structures are contained within the lungs. The right lung is divided into three lobes (upper, middle and lower) and the left lung into two lobes (upper and lower) … The structures of the chest wall (ribs, pleura, muscles of respiration) are also essential to respiration.

(Brown and Edwards, 2005, p. 544)

Example notes 1

> The respiratory system functions as a gas exchanger and is divided into the upper and lower respiratory systems.

Example notes 2

> Respiratory system (RS)
> Function – CO_2 and O_2 exchange – between blood and air
> Structure – upper respiratory tract = nose, pharynx, adenoids, tonsils, epiglottis, larynx and trachea; lower = bronchi, bronchioles, alveolar ducts and alveoli (found in lungs). Right lung = 3 lobes, Left lung = 2 lobes.

Example notes 3

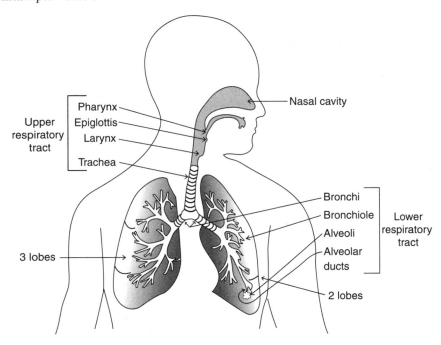

Figure 2.1 Notes from a text as an image

All of the example notes are shorter than the original paragraph. The level of detail that we take will depend on what you need/want to learn from this paragraph. The learning outcomes for the topic may help you to identify the level of detail. The notes in example 1 will remind you that there is a function and structure to the respiratory system. Example 2 notes provide further detail of the structure and I have used abbreviations where possible; '=' is my shorthand for 'consists of'. We can invent whatever abbreviations we like, so long as we remember what they mean! Example notes 3 provide both a visual aid and the detail. In Chapter 4 I will discuss with you the value of making notes using a technique called 'concept mapping' (Novak and Gowin, 1984).

It's essential to remember that making useful notes requires that you think about what you are reading and make decisions about what you will need to remember and understand. You will not need to take detailed notes of everything that you read.

Filing notes

It's useful to have at least one notebook or file on your computer in which you make your notes. It is essential to keep all of your notes together in one place so that you can find them easily when you need them. A loose-leaf folder provides the option to add pages/assignments/reports to the relevant sections of your notes. However a note pad doesn't require the discipline of keeping loose-leaf pages in order. Notes made on your computer can be easily reorganised as you need, but will need to be backed up regularly.

Accessing resources

Part of the management of your study involves accessing resources that are provided by the organisation or university at which you are enrolled. There are lots of different resources that you can access. Knowing what they are puts you in the position of being able to make an informed decision as to whether you will use these resources. In this section of the chapter I will briefly touch on two resources to consider learning about: the library and the disability office. Other resources that you may find useful to explore include counselling, computing and student services.

The disability office

If you have a disability that may impact on your studies, I encourage you to talk with your teacher, or the organisation providing your course may have a student disability office that you could contact. The disability office may be able to provide assistance such as providing specialist software, technology or equipment, course handbooks in alternative formats (e.g. audio, large print or Braille), or organise for you to have extra time to complete examinations (for example if you have dyslexia, a visual impairment or issues with manual dexterity).

The library

Even at the end of a course, some students still find the library a mystery. My strongest advice is for that *not* to be the case for you. You may well be able to access the local postgraduate centre that your primary care trust or hospital trust uses or, depending on where you are taking your course, you may be able to access the local university's library. If you can, access a library in person, take the time to familiarise yourself with the library and the resources it provides you. Almost invariably librarians are very helpful people and often with a good sense of humour.[1] They understand that initially students aren't familiar with the library. They will help you to locate the sections of the library that hold the books and journals related to the topic of your course. They will also help you to learn how to use the technology in the library, such as online catalogues, facilities for making your presentations, specialist information technology for people with disabilities, etc. Most often there are short courses, handouts or online resources on using different aspects of the library. While the organisation through which you study will have its own set of resources, the Charles Darwin University Library (Australia) has a useful podcast and transcript on locating journal articles which can be found at http://www.cdu.edu.au/library/LILL/podcasts.html.

The library will hold journals in both print and electronic formats. Very often you will find the journal information that you want through the online databases. They provide a brief description of journal articles which can help you to decide whether to read the article or not. They can be searched by subject heading and keywords. When you find an article you want to read, you may find that the database offers you a link to the full text of the article which you can read or print out straight away. However, sometimes the database will only offer you a summary of the article. If you are offered only a summary, you should check the library catalogue to find out if the full text of the article is available online or in print. Some libraries have special catalogues which cover just online journals and so you may need to check those as well. If you can't find the article you want you should ask your librarian who will be able to point you in the right direction or, if necessary, borrow the article from another library on your behalf.

In the health care field there are many databases but four of the common databases that students use are MEDLINE (via PubMed), CINAHL (Cumulative Index to Nursing and Allied Health Literature), Health Source, and the Cochrane Library. Some databases have online tutorials which provide advice on how to use their database. PubMed has animated online tutorials which describe how to search by author or subject, how to retrieve citations, and so on. Those tutorials can be found at http://www.nlm.nih.gov/bsd/disted/pubmed.html.

If you are living off campus check with your librarian or IT staff to find out if you need any special passwords or software to access databases and other university resources when you are at home.

Validity of information

Information that you find may not be valid. This means that it may not be accurate. Information on the web can be published by anyone. Generally web information is not reviewed by anyone so it may or may not be accurate. That doesn't mean you can't use and cite this information. You may need to find more than one source that says the same thing. Unlike the web, articles published in peer-reviewed journals have been reviewed by experts in the field and therefore the information in the article is therefore likely to be accurate. Books and book chapters are usually edited and the information is likely to be accurate. However a book chapter may reflect a person's opinion and as a student you need to look at the evidence that they use to support their opinion and make your own judgement about that evidence. The work that we produce for our assessments needs to be correct. We may lose marks if we use incorrect information.

Reflection and improvement

Improvement is usually part of the reason for studying. You may be studying to improve your knowledge base and/or skills. It's important to remember that studying is itself a skill and you can actively improve your study skills. So after your first week, take just a few minutes to write down your studying strengths and weaknesses as you see them (and yes, you will have strengths so do include them). Strengths may include things like: 'I can take concise notes of key ideas in readings'; or 'I am getting better at explaining important ideas I am studying to my colleagues'. Weaknesses may include things like: 'when studying I immediately look at my email any time a new message comes in'; 'I am unable to concentrate for more than five minutes at a time'; or 'I type very slowly'. Think about the things that you want to improve – try different things, talk with others about their ways of approaching these problem areas, and in a month, revisit your list and see how you are going.

Your health

As health care professionals you know the importance of sleep, exercise and diet. Maintaining your health while you study is important. You will need to read materials for your studies so it may be a good time to have your eyes checked if you have any visual problems.

Tips

1   Put aspects of study that you don't like doing with aspects that you do like doing.
2   Teaching someone else helps your own learning. Find a friend, colleague, or fellow student and explain a difficult concept to them.

The next chapter

The following chapter explores what learning is, identifies different learning outcomes and discusses different learning strategies from which students can choose. The chapter focuses on helping students see that there are choices to be made about how we learn and that we need to be strategic about our learning.

3 Learning

Learning outcomes

By the end of this chapter readers are expected to be able to:

- identify different types of learning outcomes
- identify and select different strategies or ways of learning
- evaluate the usefulness of various ways of learning in different situations and contexts, and
- appreciate that learners need to be strategic in the ways that they learn.

Introduction

There are many ways of learning and different strategies to help us learn. The intention of this chapter is to show you that there isn't one right way to learn. A way of learning that works in one context may not be as useful in another context. We have choices about how we learn and we are in a strong position if we know what those choices are so that we can make informed decisions.

You may have heard references to 'learning styles'. You have probably heard people talking about visual, auditory or kinaesthetic learners. Honey and Mumford (1992) identified four categories of learners: activist, pragmatist, reflector and theorist; while Kolb and Fry (1975) identified four different learning styles: converger, diverger, accommodator and assimilator (Kolb, 1984). The focus of this chapter is not on learning styles because I don't find 'learning styles' to be a particularly helpful way of thinking about learning. This chapter will focus on what I do believe will help you to be a better learner and if you do want to find out more about learning styles, it is easy to do a web search to find websites that discuss the different types. This chapter discusses:

- what learning is
- how teachers teach to help students to learn
- how students can take advantage of the learning opportunities that their teachers provide
- the four domains of learning, and
- seven elements of learning (or strategies for learning).

I anticipate that some of the ideas in this chapter will be new to you while other ideas may be a refresher. I am sure that many if not all of the ideas discussed in the chapter can help you to improve your learning. Figure 3.1 provides a concept map that summarises my view of the key ideas in this chapter and how I think that those ideas are interlinked. Don't worry if you don't understand all of the terms in the figure as they will be explained later in this chapter. As you look at Figure 3.1 you will see that I believe that teachers foster student learning by using good teaching practices, that learning can be categorised into four different categories called domains; that students can use seven different elements or strategies to help them learn and that those elements can help students to learn in the different domains.

What is learning?

I believe that having an image[1] of what learning is may help us to learn. So I am going to share with you what I think learning 'looks like'. I like to think of learning as making connections in my head. If you think of your mind as a very complex Meccano set or intricate scaffolding, learning occurs when we:

1   introduce new pieces into the mind and connect them to pieces that are already there
2   we make new connections between separate pieces that were already in our mind, or
3   introduce separate, new pieces into the mind in a group but don't connect them to anything that is already there and we may not necessarily connect the new pieces to each other either (Ausubel, 1968; Novak and Gowin, 1984).

I envisage this last way as the way that we first learn something 'off by heart'. That's not to say that over time these new pieces of information won't be connected to other concepts already in our heads, but that takes effort and time. Figure 3.2 illustrates learning for meaning (assimilation) and memorising or learning by rote. In the illustration on the left-hand side the three pieces of new information aren't connected to the existing ideas in the mind. This sort of learning represents rote learning. In the illustration on the right-hand side, the three new pieces of information are connected to ideas that already exist in the mind. This is called meaningful learning or assimilation.

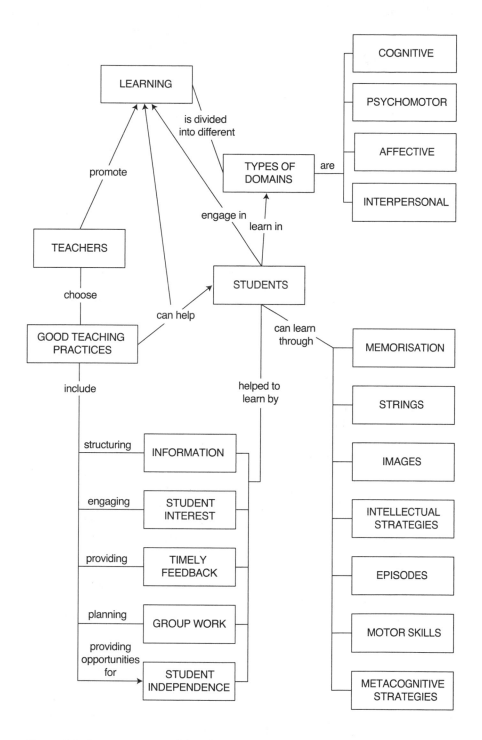

Figure 3.1 A concept map of the ideas about learning discussed in this chapter

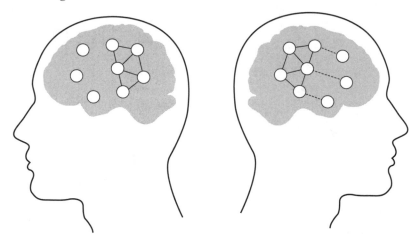

Figure 3.2 Learning by rote and learning for meaning. The illustration on the left-hand side represents new information learnt by rote while the illustration on the right-hand side represents new information learnt through assimilation with existing knowledge

The 'pieces' are ideas or concepts and are represented by nouns. The 'connections' are most often verbs (Novak and Gowin, 1984). So for example, two concepts are 'sky' and 'blue'. When I lived in Australia the way I connected those two concepts together to make sense of them was 'The sky is blue'. When I lived in the UK, to make sense of these concepts I needed to change that connection to 'The sky is sometimes blue'![2]

I want to use this image of learning to illustrate the difference between 'knowledge' and 'information'. Teachers, books, the web, television and so on can provide us with information. We then turn that information into knowledge and we do that by taking the information into our minds and making sense of it. This next piece is really important for learners. Individuals construct knowledge and make sense of information by making those connections in their minds (Bruner, 1990; Novak, 1993; Sherman, 1995). I believe that this is important for every student to understand because it means that the responsibilities of teachers and students are very different. They have very different jobs to do.

The student's job is to learn and only the student is responsible for his or her own learning.

The teacher's job is to design opportunities and environments in which students can learn. Teachers can help students to learn, but at the end of the day the student is responsible for his or her own learning. Having made this distinction between student and teacher responsibilities I'd like to explore with you some of the ways in which you can take advantage of the things that teachers do to help their students to learn.

Ways teachers help students to learn

I'd like you to think about one or two teachers who taught you in secondary school or post secondary school, who you think really helped you to learn. Before you turn the page try to make a list of the things that you think they did or how they were that helped you to learn. Can you think of six or seven things?

Chances are your list includes things such as: was enthusiastic about the topic; cared about the students; could make complex ideas simple; was a good communicator; respected students' opinions; returned my assignments promptly and made helpful comments; used humour; valued what I had to say; and made it clear what students needed to achieve. I'd like to explore some of these ideas a little further because I believe that by being aware of what good teachers do to help learning, students may be better prepared to take advantage of their teachers' efforts. In the following pages I discuss five good teaching practices that teachers use to help students to learn. I could have chosen six or ten or twenty different good teaching practices. I've chosen five to provide you with a variety of ideas and a starting point. Once you look for these five in your courses, you will be able to identify other good teaching practices and think about how to use them to your benefit. The five good teaching practices that I have chosen are:

1   structuring the information that they are teaching
2   engaging student interest
3   providing student independence and control in their studies
4   providing timely and useful feedback, and
5   helping students to work in groups.

These five practices are drawn from two different sources and my own experience of teaching over many years (HERDSA, 1992; Center for Teaching Effectiveness, 2008). I will discuss each practice in turn and provide suggestions for how you might try to learn when your teachers use them.

Structure

Teachers provide students with lots of information and rather than provide that information as individual pieces, they often try to organise the information into a structure, to group similar ideas together and to show the ways in which different ideas fit together. They do this to help students organise the information and to develop the information into knowledge in their minds. Teachers demonstrate a structure in their teaching in at least three different ways and perhaps you can think of others:

1   by organising the topics they are going to talk about and providing a clear and structured outline or agenda that is easy for students to follow. The teacher is trying to provide students with a 'road map' of what to expect and where s/he hopes students will be at the end of the session
2   by using 'signposts' in the teaching session to show what the session has covered and how the next topic links with the last topic, and
3   by drawing links between a session and information in previous sessions (lectures/tutorials/laboratory sessions/seminars/online discussions and exercises).

There are at least two things that students can do to take advantage of these teaching approaches. First pay close attention to the learning outcomes. When you review the session, check to see if you think that you can demonstrate all of the learning outcomes. If you are not sure whether you can or can't, you can always talk with the teacher to see what exactly would be required for you to demonstrate particular learning outcomes. Please don't worry that you are asking silly questions. In my experience teachers are delighted to know that students are taking note of the learning outcomes that the teacher has prepared. They want you to succeed.

The second thing that you can do during the session is try to keep the agenda for the whole session in front of you. Pay attention to when new topics are started and what the teacher said as s/he moved from one topic to the next. If it's not clear to you how or if one topic is linked to the next, you can always ask the teacher if they are linked. Making those connections between different topic areas can really help students to make sense of different sets of information.

Engagement and interest

Generally teachers are interested in the topic that they are teaching and they want you to share that interest. They are aware that being interested in a topic provides students with an intrinsic motivation to learn and understand the topic. There are many ways in which student interest in a topic can be stimulated. You can probably identify several ways if you think back to some of the good teachers who have taught you over the years. They probably used analogies and stories, they personalised their teaching by bringing in their own experiences of the topic, they used a variety of different activities during the teaching sessions (such as demonstrations, slides, video, role play, etc.) and they showed that they were interested in and enthusiastic about the subject matter. The teacher may try to make the course relevant to students by drawing connections and relationships between your working context and the course information and to do so you may be asked to bring an example or a patient case from your workplace.

There are a number of things that you as a student can do to take advantage of these teaching approaches.

- Teachers aren't the only ones who can think of analogies to help make sense of an idea. Students can too. There is nothing to stop you and your fellow students thinking of analogies to help to explain topics, and
- Some topics lend themselves to 'real life' in that they can be identified in work situations or the media. As a student you can try to identify 'real life' examples of topics discussed in your classes.

Can you think of any other ways in which you can make the ideas more real and engaging?

Student independence and control

As students if we have some sense of control or independence in our courses we can be more motivated to learn and the learning can be more meaningful (Ramsden, 2003). If your course has been designed to provide you with choice, I suggest that you make the best use of the opportunity. For example, for assessment purposes you may be required to write an assignment in which you can choose some elements, whether the topic, or the approach you take to a particular topic. Therefore it can be useful to think about what you would find most interesting or valuable. Can you make this assignment relevant to your work practice (for example by developing a teaching session on a health issue or doing an audit or review of your workplace to identify changes in practice or identify a service need)? If you can, you will be achieving three things with the one effort: 1) completing an assessment for your course; 2) contributing to your everyday work and 3) doing something in which you have an interest and are personally invested. Alternatively you may be able to take a particular approach to an assessment that would give you valuable experience: for example, interviewing people; designing a concept map or a mind map; developing a work plan; etc.

Feedback

Ramsden (2003) writes that on a course experience questionnaire he designed, the question 'that differentiated most effectively between the best and the worst courses ... was concerned with the quality of feedback on students' progress' (p. 96). 'Of all the facets of teaching that are important to [students], feedback on assessed work is perhaps the most commonly mentioned' (p. 96).

As students we are rightly concerned with assessment. Assessment requirements provide us with the opportunity to demonstrate what we have learnt during the course. Some students don't make the best use of teacher feedback. It can be invaluable to future learning to pay very close attention to the feedback you receive on your work. Just looking at the mark or grade probably isn't going to give you much information about how to improve your next piece of assessment. Rereading your assessment in light of the teacher's comments may well give you insights into how to improve the next assessment. If you're not sure, go and talk with your teacher, another student or a colleague about your work. Very few students talk with their teachers about the feedback on their assessments. Many teachers welcome the opportunity to talk with students about their work. One very useful question to ask your teacher is if s/he could suggest particular things that you could do to improve your work for your next assessment (e.g. having someone read a draft before you submit the assignment). Reflecting on your assessment is an important element in your learning.

Cooperating with and learning from other students

Learning is enhanced when it is more like a team effort than a solo race. Good learning, like good work, is collaborative and social, not competitive and isolated. Working with others often increases involvement in learning. Sharing one's own ideas and responding to others' reactions improves thinking and deepens understanding.

(The Seven Principles Resource Center, adapted in Center for Teaching Effectiveness, 2008)

Group work is a process of learning that simulates professional practice. This process helps students to develop further essential interpersonal skills for working effectively in teams in the future. Participating in group work highlights group dynamics and processes and requires empathy and understanding, all of which help to build better teamwork. Group work allows individuals to share ideas and experiences which will be an essential part of your professional development into the future.

Your teacher may or may not organise for students to work in groups and even when they do, some students may not take full advantage of the opportunity. Sometimes students think that the only sources of valid information are the teacher and the textbook. It would be a mistake not to make the most of working with other students. If your teacher hasn't organised you into groups there is nothing to stop you from asking several others on the course if they'd like to work with you in a study group. You don't necessarily have to meet face to face in order to work in a group. You can meet online or over the phone.

Group work is so important that Chapter 8 is completely dedicated to the topic. The authors of Chapter 8 have also developed a website about group work which you might find useful. This website discusses group processes and issues such as group brainstorming, making decisions, planning, giving and receiving feedback, working well together and conflict management (http://www.griffith.edu.au/cgi-bin/frameit?http://www.griffith.edu.au/school/hsv/content/assistance/guides_skills/assistance_guides_group_work.html).

To conclude, in this section on 'Ways teachers help students to learn' we've discussed five ways in which teachers use good teaching principles and practices to help students to learn. By knowing these teaching principles and some of the practices that teachers use, students can capitalise on them. Now I'd like to move from strategies to use to take advantage of good teaching principles to discuss with you four different areas (domains) of learning: cognitive, psychomotor skills, affective and interpersonal communication.

Domains of learning

I believe that it can be very helpful for learners to identify what they are trying to achieve when they are learning about a topic. What is the desired learning outcome? Knowing this can guide the ways you can choose to learn which we will explore in the next section of this chapter, 'Elements of learning'. To explore this further I'd like to introduce you to the four 'domains of learning':

1   cognitive domain: intellectual abilities and skills
2   psychomotor domain: hand–eye coordination, motor skills, manual dexterity, etc.
3   affective domain: developing feelings, attitudes, values and ethics, and
4   interpersonal domain: interpersonal skills, communication skills, listening skills, ability to work as a team member, leadership skills, etc.

The learning outcomes or objectives of a course let students know on which domains of learning the course focuses. Predominantly courses focus on learning outcomes in the cognitive domain and that's the domain that we will discuss in this chapter. The idea for the cognitive or intellectual domain was first put forward in 1956 by Benjamin Bloom. He identified six outcomes of learning in the cognitive domain. Table 3.1 illustrates those six outcomes and you can see from the table that in the cognitive domain people can recall, comprehend, apply, analyse, synthesise or evaluate information. There is a hierarchy associated with Bloom's cognitive domain, with synthesis and evaluation being more demanding than recall and comprehension. In higher education courses learners can expect to be asked to demonstrate their understanding through all elements of the hierarchy.

Table 3.1 Six types of learning outcomes in the cognitive domain (Bloom, 1956)

Learning type	*Examples*
Recall or recognise	Terminology, facts, definitions, conventions, trends, sequences, classification categories, criteria, methodologies, principles, generalisations, theories and structures
Comprehension	Paraphrase, summarise, extrapolate, interpret, select, explain, classify, translate
Application	Predict, problem solve, calculate, perform
Analysis	Of both content and form – identify elements, determine relationships/connections between components, check consistency, determine organising structures, compare and contrast, justify, interpret relationships
Synthesis	Put together elements in a way that wasn't evident before, compose, propose, derive, design
Evaluation	Judgements about the value of something for a given purpose, find fallacies, assess accuracy, consistency, compare and choose, apply criteria and choose, interpret evidence, argue argue for and against

What does distinguishing between those six learning outcomes in the cognitive domain mean for students? Knowing about these six learning outcomes helps us to decide what we want to do with the information that we are studying. These outcomes can also help us to decipher the learning outcomes that the teacher has identified for the course. For example, you may decide that the best way to learn the twelve cranial nerves (olfactory, optic, oculomotor, trochlear, trigeminal, abducens, facial, auditory [vestibulo-cochlear], glossopharyngeal, vagus, spinal accessory, hypoglossal) is to memorise (recall) them. On the other hand, you may decide that the best way to learn how to titrate insulin is to observe and work through particular situations in a diabetes clinic. Whatever you choose, you need to keep in mind at least three things: 1) what learning does the teacher want you to do? 2) what type of learning (memorisation, evaluation, etc.) does the assessment require you to demonstrate? and 3) what do you want to learn from this course?

We have discussed in this chapter the different types of learning in the cognitive domain because most academic courses focus on learning through the cognitive domain. If your course has an emphasis on psychomotor skills or affective (values) outcomes you may find the following website useful: 'Learning domains or Bloom's taxonomy': http://www.nwlink.com/~donclark/hrd/bloom.html.

In this section of the chapter we have touched on different types of learning domains and learning outcomes. In the next section I want to explore with you different ways of learning, which White and Gunstone (1992) refer to as different elements of learning.

Elements of learning

Over your lifetime you have spent many thousands of hours learning for formal education. What I'd like you to do now is to take out a piece of paper and take a few minutes to think about and list the sorts of things that you do when you want to learn something – e.g. make notes. Can you list four or five other things?

When I ask students this question they tell me the following sorts of things: reading, listening, writing, memorising, making notes, solving problems, discussing in groups, practising, role play, and so on. All of these are ways that we can use to learn and we can improve our effectiveness in each of these ways over time with thought and practice. In the last section of this chapter I'd like to introduce you to some ideas about student learning that you may not have come across before. The ideas are called the 'seven elements of learning' and they come from the work of two academics from Monash University.

The seven elements of learning (White and Gunstone, 1992)

I'd like to demonstrate these ideas by giving you a test. It's not important that you get the answers right. I'm using the test to demonstrate the seven elements or ways of learning. I would like you to take out a piece of paper and answer the following seven questions. I believe that the ideas will have more of an impact on you if you try to answer the questions before looking at the answers.

Question 1 What is the national capital of Canada?

Question 2 Finish this sentence: 'A stitch in time ...'

Question 3 Draw a Bunsen burner.

Question 4 Write about the last time you saw blood (which isn't menstrual blood).

Question 5 Solve this algorithm: $4x + 2 = 0$.

Question 6 How did you learn to do an aseptic handwash?

Question 7 Think of the last exam that you did. If you had to do that exam again name one thing that you'd do to improve the result of that exam.

Explanations of the test

Question 1

The answer is 'Ottawa'. This is a fact and either you know it or you don't. Unless you have been to Ottawa, the way to learn this fact is to **memorise** it. Memorising facts is one element or way of learning.

Question 2

The answer is 'A stitch in time saves nine'. This element of learning is called a '**string**'. The saying means that doing something now (like mending a small hole in a shirt) will save a lot more work and time than if we do the work later, i.e. if the hole is left to get bigger. Strings help us to store lots of information. For example 'Roy G Biv' and 'Richard of York gave battle in vain' are strings that help students to learn the colours of the rainbow and their order (red, orange, yellow, green, blue, indigo, violet). Another example of a string is 'On old Olympus towering tops a Fin and German viewed some hops' which students use to remember the twelve cranial nerves. Using strings is the second element of learning.

Question 3

'**Images**' are White and Gunstone's third element of learning. We can learn about something, in this case a Bunsen burner, by using our sensory perceptions to visualise the equipment. The image helps us to develop our knowledge about the equipment and how it is set up (Figure 3.3). Smell, touch, taste and sound are the other sensory perceptions that we can use to learn about something. For example, we can learn a lot about heart beats by listening to them.

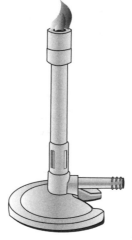

Figure 3.3 An image of a Bunsen burner

Question 4

White and Gunstone call their fourth element of learning '**episodes**'. An episode is the memory of an event. The learning is put into a context, feelings as well as sensory perceptions are incorporated and this often results in very powerful learning. An Australian friend of mine was using a chainsaw to cut timber on his rural property when the timber he was cutting gave way unexpectedly and the chainsaw cut into the calf of his leg. This experience was a very powerful learning episode for him. Amongst other things he learnt to wear chain mail protective gear when using the chainsaw. Perhaps you can think of something that you learned through an 'episode' in which context, feelings and sensory perceptions contributed to your learning. I expect that health care professionals can learn a great deal the first time they have to break bad news to a patient or the family of a patient.

Question 5

The answer to question 5 is $-\frac{1}{2}$ or -0.5

$$4x + 2 = 0$$
$$4x = -2$$
$$x = -\tfrac{2}{4}$$
$$x = -\tfrac{1}{2} \text{ or } -0.5$$

This is an algorithm, which is an **intellectual strategy**. It's the recall of a procedure or application. We have to use the right intellectual strategy in the right context. For example when we want to calculate a person's body mass index (BMI) we need to know that the formula is weight (kg)/height^2 (m^2). So the intellectual strategy used in the calculation of body mass index requires two steps: first the conversion of height from centimetres into metres (e.g. 165 cm = 165/100 m = 1.65 m) and then the division of weight in kilograms by the height in metres squared. So a 70 kg person of 165 cm has a BMI of 25.7 (70/1.65 × 1.65).

Question 6

Most people say that they learnt to do an aseptic handwash by watching someone do it and then practising the procedure, with constructive feedback (watch one, try one, do one). This is a **motor skill** and most if not all motor skills are best learnt by doing them, preferably combined with constructive feedback.

Question 7

When I ask students this question they have a lot of different answers: not stay up all night cramming; not stay up drinking the night before; read several past exam papers; read the questions more carefully, etc. Whatever your answer, what you are doing is demonstrating that you can reflect on your learning and make changes to improve it. This element of learning is called a **metacognitive strategy**. Many students don't think about how they learn and it's very difficult if not impossible to improve how we learn if we don't reflect on our learning.

The seven elements are seven ways in which to learn about something. No one element that White and Gunstone (1992) propose is necessarily better than any of the others. They argue that the more elements a learner uses, the more likely it is that their understanding of that topic will be better than if they learnt about it only using one way.

The very next time you set out to learn about a topic, you might find it useful first to think about which of the above elements you will use. Will you: memorise the facts about the topic; use a string or motor skills or your sensory perceptions or an intellectual strategy; try to experience the topic through a particular context? During your course will you set aside the time to think about how you are learning and if you could improve the ways in which you are learning?

So far in this chapter we have explored:

- what learning looks like (linking ideas to other ideas in your mind)
- strategies to use to take advantage of some of your teachers' good teaching practices (providing structure of the information that they are teaching; engaging student interest; providing timely and useful feedback; helping students to work in groups; and providing student independence and control in their courses)
- different types of learning outcomes (recall/recognition, comprehension, application, analysis, synthesis and evaluation), and
- different ways of learning (memorisation, strings, images, episodes, intellectual strategy, motor skill, metacognitive strategy).

Tips

1   Teachers are a fantastic resource and surprisingly few students avail themselves of the opportunity to talk with their teachers. Make the time to discuss your work with your teachers, or another student or work colleague.

2   Sometimes it might be useful to memorise some information, while at other times we may need to understand and be able to apply certain concepts. As students we are expected to be strategic. Deciding when you are going to memorise and when you are going to try to make sense of a topic is being strategic.

3   'Learning is not a spectator sport. Students do not learn much just sitting in classes listening to the teacher, memorizing information, and reproducing answers. They must talk about what they are learning, write about it, relate it to past experiences, and apply it to their daily lives' (Chickering and Gamson, 1987, pp. 3–7).

The next chapter

Making links between new information and the existing knowledge in our mind helps us to understand the new information. In the following chapter I will discuss a technique that can help us to make those links in our minds. The technique is called concept mapping.

4 Concept mapping
A strategy to make meaning

Learning outcomes

By the end of this chapter readers are expected to be able to:

- construct a concept map
- identify when it would be helpful to use concept maps, and
- use different ways to improve your concept maps.

Introduction

In Chapter 3 I suggested that learning consists of making connections between ideas in our minds and that we make these connections by introducing new ideas and connecting them to ideas that are already in our minds or by making new connections between the ideas already there. Concept mapping is a technique that people use to help them make those connections. I have found that many students find making concept maps extremely helpful when learning new topics and I have devoted this chapter to showing you how to make concept maps and how to use them when studying (Fraser and Edwards, 1985). In this chapter I will discuss what concept maps are, how making them can help you to learn, how to construct them, what to look for in your maps in order to improve them and how to use them in lectures, writing assignments, studying for exams, etc.

Introduction to concept maps

Concept maps were developed in 1974 by Novak and his students and have been used in many countries throughout the world. A concept map is a diagram that is like a road map in that it 'not only identifies the major points of interest (concepts), but also illustrates the relationships among the concepts in much the same way that links among cities are illustrated by highways and other roads' (Novak, 1980, pp. III–1). If you refer to Figure 4.1 you will see

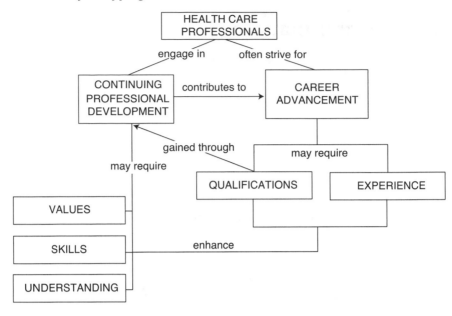

Figure 4.1 An example of a concept map, illustrating some of the characteristics of a concept map

that the words in the boxes are the 'concepts'. These are generally nouns. The words on the lines between the concepts are linking words, often verbs, and they explain the relationship between the concepts; they make the relationship make sense. Two concepts are linked to create what Novak refers to as a proposition (Novak and Gowin, 1984). 'Continuing professional development contributes to career advancement' is a proposition in which two concepts, 'continuing professional development' and 'career advancement', are linked together by the linking words 'contributes to', to create meaning. The person making the concept map could change the meaning by writing 'Continuing professional development does not contribute to career advancement'. The person making the map shows their understanding by the linking words that they use and by which concepts they link together.

Before describing concept maps, I want to demonstrate the difference between a concept map, a mind map and a flow chart. This next section of the chapter is a direct quote from a guide that I wrote for university teachers in 1996 (Fraser, 1996). The ideas are directly relevant to you as a university student. Please note that in the quote, the content of square brackets, [], denotes changes from the original text.

MIND MAPS, FLOW CHARTS AND CONCEPT MAPS:
A COMPARISON

Some people, when first introduced to the technique of concept mapping, initially believe that they have 'done this' before because they have experienced using the techniques of mind mapping or flow chart-ing. At first glance the techniques may appear similar. To demonstrate the differences between these three techniques, a flow chart, mind map and concept map of the topic 'Concept Maps' are represented respec-tively in Figures [4.2, 4.3 and 4.4].

A flow chart focuses on the procedures of the task at hand, which, in Figure [4.2], is the task of constructing a concept map. It represents what Gagne refers to as procedural knowledge [in which the process is described], specifying the sequential actions to be carried out and the decisions to be made at certain points in the process (Gagne, 1985). While it is useful in some circumstances to be able to delineate the sequential actions within a process, in tertiary education we are also concerned with the student's ability to demonstrate conceptual under-standing. Both mind maps and concept maps primarily incorporate conceptual information although procedural information can be included in both.

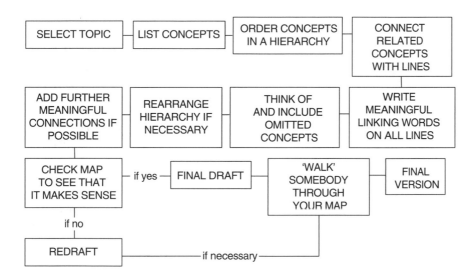

Figure 4.2 A flow chart of the topic 'concept maps'. A flow chart specifies the sequential actions to be carried out and the decisions to be made at certain points in the process of constructing a concept map (Fraser, 1996, p. 17)

Mind maps, Figure 4.3, incorporate conceptual associations. Buzan sug-gests that 'if the brain works primarily with key concepts in an interlinked and integrated manner, our notes and our word relations should in many instances be structured in this way rather than in tradi-tional "lines"' (Buzan, 1983, p. 91). The centre of a mind map incorporates an image of the central idea of the topic. Images may also be used in other parts of the map. From this central image the individual draws a line and on that line writes another idea (concept) which she associates with the central image. This second idea is then associated with another and so forth until that stream is exhausted. The individual returns to the central image and begins again. Although mind maps do not begin at the top of the page and work their way down, they do represent a hierarchy as the 'more important ideas will be nearer the centre and the less important ideas will be near the edge' (Buzan, 1983 p. 92). [In Figure 4.3 the central image is of our topic 'concept maps'. On the top line I have added the following ideas that I associate with the image of concept maps; 'hierarchy', 'context', 'most specific concept' and 'most inclusive concept'. Then I started the second line on my mind map, again starting at the central image of the concept map.]

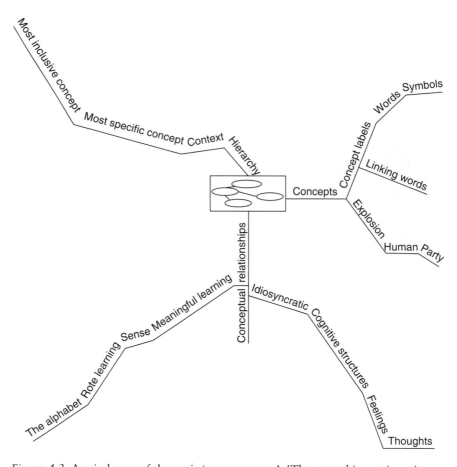

Figure 4.3 A mind map of the topic 'concept maps'. [The central image is an image of a concept map] (Fraser, 1996, p. 18)

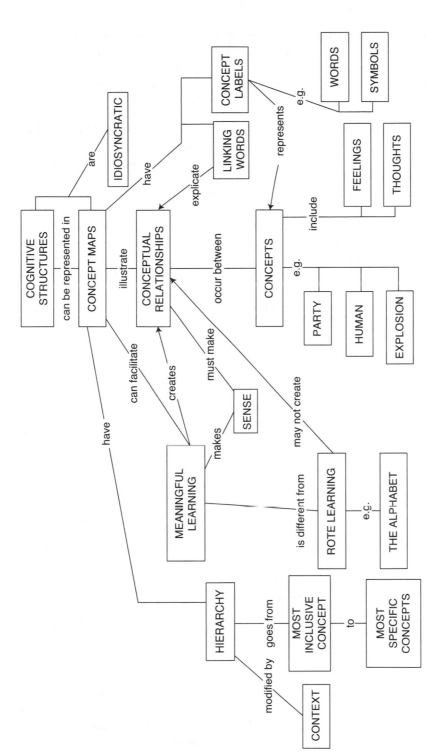

Figure 4.4 A concept map of the topic 'concept maps' (Fraser, 1996, p. 19)

Identical concepts have been incorporated into both the mind map in Figure [4.3] and the concept map in Figure [4.4]. Unlike the mind map, the concept map explicitly states the meaning of the relationship between each pair of linked concepts. The concept map clearly depicts what the author understands about the topic of 'Concept Maps'. This is not the case with the mind map. The mind map indicates only what concepts the author associates with the topic of 'Concept Maps'. It does not indicate the meaning constructed about the topic.

(Fraser, 1996, pp. 16–17)

A concept map helps students to make sense of the topic in ways that flow-charts and mind maps can't. Concept maps can be used to help you to study. Having compared concept maps, flowcharts and mind maps, I will further introduce you to concept maps by describing their characteristics. The section 'Characteristics of a Concept Map' is a direct quote from my previous work (Fraser, 1996); however the concept maps are new and have been constructed specifically for this book. The content of square brackets [] again denotes changes from the original text.

CHARACTERISTICS OF A CONCEPT MAP
There are several characteristics to note in the construction of a concept map.

1   The structure is hierarchical, with more inclusive, general concepts [such as 'health care professionals' in Figure 4.1] placed at the top of the map and less inclusive, specific concepts [such as 'skills' in Figure 4.1] placed toward the bottom of the map. Each concept may be enclosed in a rectangle or other geometric form. Lines are drawn to connect the concepts. Linking words which explain the nature of the relationship between each pair of concepts are written on the lines. These characteristics are illustrated in Figures [4.1, 4.5 and 4.6].
2   Linking words should always exist on the lines that connect concepts. The linkages themselves should consist of one or only a few words. The linking words specifically explain the relationship between the concepts. In the example 'The sky is blue', 'is' is the linking word. Linking words do not form a sentence by themselves.
3   Concept maps flow from the top to the bottom of the page. Arrows need only be used to indicate the direction of the relationship when it is not from top to bottom. Notice where arrows are used in Figures [4.1, 4.5 and 4.6].
4   A concept map represents an individual's understanding of a topic. Different people may understand the same topic slightly differently and therefore produce different maps. One map can be as valid as the next, and there is no one 'right' map. This is illustrated in Figure [4.6] in which the same set of concepts is mapped in two different maps. It

must be noted that although two maps containing the same concepts may be different and equally valid, it is possible for one map to contain faulty propositions and therefore not be as valid as another.

5 The power of a concept map derives from the interconnections between and among the concepts. Increasing the number of meaningful cross-linkages in different sections of the map indicates an increasingly sophisticated level of understanding on the part of the individual. Compare the two maps in Figure [4.8].

6 Feelings can be expressed on a concept map by including concepts such as fear, anger, enjoyment, fulfillment, stress, etc., and by choosing more emphatic linking words. Part of the meaning that we create from our experiences includes affective connotations, and these also need to be included in the concept map. Refer to Figure [4.9]. Including the concept 'stress' adds an important perspective to [the] figure. Whether learning new material or reconceptualising familiar material, the concept mapping process allows the individual to visually represent her cognitive structure and see her web of interconnected conceptual meanings. In constructing a map the individual is able to represent and ascertain the specific understanding that she holds about a certain topic or event. Through the actual process of constructing a concept map, the individual can also make new connections and recognise concepts which need to be included. While a concept map cannot provide 'a definitive picture of the realities of the situation', concept mapping can be used to assist an individual to structure her own understanding of a topic and to create personal meaning (Symington and Novak, 1982, p. 16).

(Fraser, 1996, pp. 11–15)

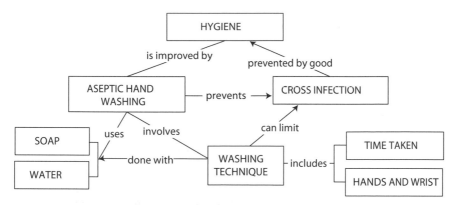

Figure 4.5 This concept map about improving hygiene through aseptic hand washing demonstrates that while concept maps flow from top to bottom, arrows can be used to indicate the direction of the relationship when it is not from top to bottom

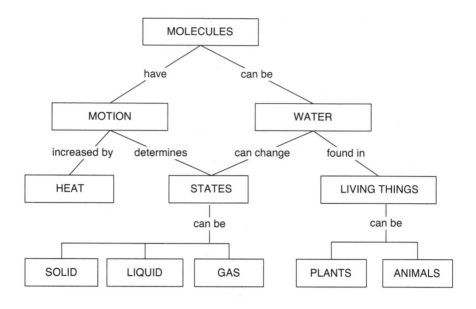

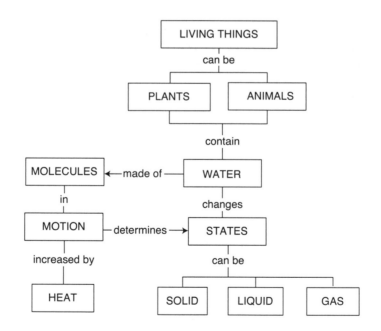

Figure 4.6 Creating two different but valid concept maps containing the same
concepts, Novak and Gowin (1984, p. 18) illustrated that no one map
is 'correct'. A concept map represents the individual's understanding of
the topic, and unless the understanding includes misconceptions, the
map is valid (Fraser, 1996, p. 13)

Constructing a concept map

The map that you construct represents the way in which you understand the concepts. Connecting concepts requires time, effort and thought. As before, this next section is a direct quote from my previous work.

> As a general rule an individual will need to do several drafts of each map. When constructing maps, some people use a pencil and use their eraser liberally; some put the concepts on 'post its' and move them around; some construct their maps using computer programmes (ABC Flow Charter, [Winflow] and MacFlow are two examples of programmes that can be used to create concept maps). Your mapping technique will improve rapidly with practice. There isn't one 'right' way to construct a concept map.
>
> ONE OPTION FOR CONSTRUCTING A CONCEPT MAP
>
> 1   The first time you construct a concept map, keep it simple and small. Begin by selecting a relatively simple topic with which you are familiar. Identify and list 6–10 relevant concepts. Remember that 'concepts' are different from 'linking words'. Concepts are events, things that happen (eg. a party, training) or objects, anything that exists and can be observed (eg. a chair, a text). Remember that you can include affective concepts [feelings and values].
>
> 2   Having selected the relevant concepts, there are at least two different ways to approach actually mapping the concepts. Some people choose to evaluate the relative importance of the concepts they've selected, ranking them from the most inclusive to the least inclusive. Then they arrange the concepts in clusters and draw in and label the connecting lines. Other people choose to select the most inclusive concept for the 'heading' of the map. Without ranking the rest of the concepts, they select the concepts that relate most directly to the 'heading' and then select concepts that most closely relate to those concepts already on the map. Choose whichever way works for you to develop your initial hierarchy. As you connect the concepts make sure that you write linking words on all of the lines connecting concepts to each other. Linking words make sense of the relationships between concepts. They are not concepts. Some examples of linking words are: consist of, form, are, with, identifies.
>
> 3   Take another look at the hierarchy that you have chosen and see if it makes sense to you. Perhaps you will choose to move one or more concepts further up or down or to the sides of your map.
>
> 4   Look to see if you can create further meaningful connections between concepts on your map. Pay attention to the concepts on the side edges and the concepts at the top and bottom of the map.

Are there meaningful relationships that can be drawn between concepts on these edges?

5   At this stage it may be useful to include more concepts on your map. In so doing it may be necessary for you to reorganise the hierarchy.

6   'Walk' somebody else through your draft map. It may be most useful to choose someone who is not familiar with the topic of your map. This will help you to make sure that the connections you have chosen really do make sense.

CREATING THE INITIAL LIST OF CONCEPTS

Sometimes the list of concepts to be included in your map is predetermined because of the task that you are doing. For instance, if you are summarising a journal article, then you will select what you consider to be the key concepts in the article and map the interrelationships that the author makes. However, sometimes we begin with a blank sheet of paper and a heading. Creating the list of concepts to map can be achieved in a number of ways, including:

1   Brain storming a comprehensive list with or without the assistance of others;
2   Adding concepts to your map as you construct it; and
3   Mind mapping the topic (Buzan, 1983).

(Fraser, 1996, pp. 22–24)

Remember that you can always add concepts to or subtract concepts from your map. Whether you construct a list of concepts first or whether you move straight to constructing your map, the important thing is to start.

What to look for in your concept maps

When you have drafted your map you can review it to see if you can improve it. Here are several things which you can look for when reviewing your map (adapted from Fraser, 1996).

1   Missing linking words: The omission of words on a line linking two concepts will occur more often than you may anticipate. If you have drawn a line between two concepts and you don't know what words to write on the line, you may need to go back to your text, notes, the web, etc. to find out exactly what the concepts mean and to see if you can link them sensibly.

2   Linking 'sentences': Instead of writing a few linking words you may have written linking sentences. It's likely that there are concepts in these sentences (i.e. nouns). If there are, identify the concepts on the lines and separate them out as concepts in boxes. Now try to link your

new concepts into your map and remember: try to use very few linking words to illustrate the relationships. In the top map of Figure 4.7 the concept of 'professional development' is included in the linking words between the concepts 'new roles' and 'patient treatment'. Making 'professional development' a clearly separate concept creates a different relationship between the concepts of 'new roles' and 'patient treatment', as shown in the bottom map of Figure 4.7.

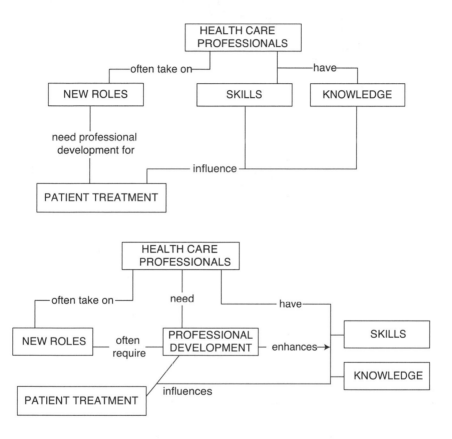

Figure 4.7 Concepts on linking lines

3   A straight line map: A straight line map is basically a sentence with no cross-linkages. Refer to Figure 4.8. Linking concepts to each other allows you to show what you understand the concepts to mean. If your concept map has very few lines between concepts, look to see if you can include more lines between the boxes. You may need to do some more work to understand what the concepts mean and what they mean in relation to each other. In particular look for relationships between concepts on the

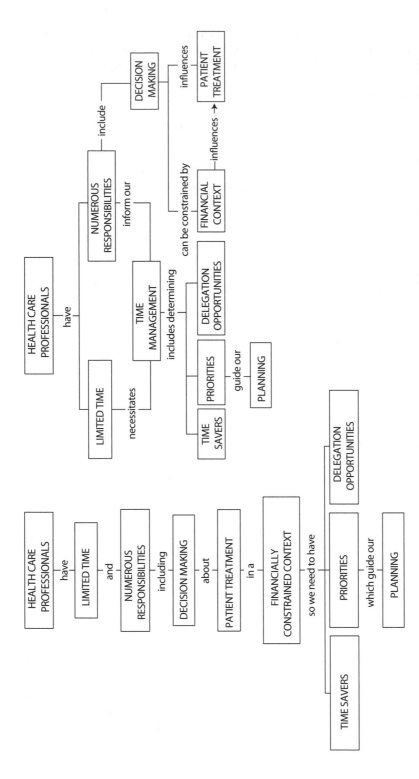

Figure 4.8 The power of a concept map is derived from the interconnections constructed between and among the concepts. The left map is a 'straight line' map which could just as easily be written in a paragraph. The right map incorporates interconnections between and among the concepts

two side edges of the page and between concepts at the top and bottom of the map. If you do find that you can link these concepts, you may need to reorganise where your concepts fit on your map.

4   Misconceptions: It's possible that in your map you have represented misconceptions and misunderstandings that you hold. Asking your teacher, colleague or another student to read some of your maps may help you to identify and then change your misconceptions. It can be much easier for someone else to spot a misconception in a concept map than in a page of notes. It also takes very little time for someone to read a concept map compared with a page of notes.

5   Omitted concepts: You may not be able to fit a concept meaningfully into your map. Further study of the concept may be necessary in order to do so. Perhaps on the side of your map list those concepts that seem relevant to the topic but that you can't fit into your map. Later you may be able to find out more about those concepts in order to include them or you may be able to ask someone else how they would fit them into your map.

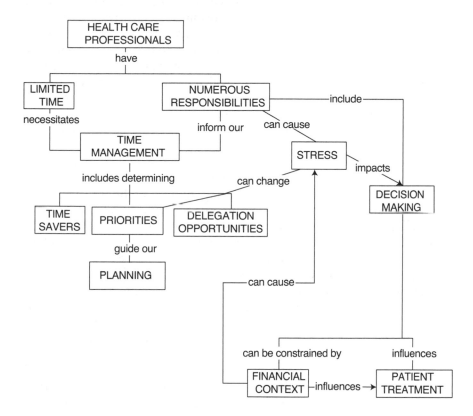

Figure 4.9 The inclusion of feelings and values can be usefully incorporated into concept maps. Including the concept 'stress' adds an important perspective to this map

6   Non-meaningful linkages: In your map each individual proposition (two concepts linked together) must make sense. For example 'The sky is blue' makes sense by itself. In the left map of Figure 4.8, the proposition 'limited time and numerous responsibilities' does not mean anything by itself. The right map of Figure 4.8 has reorganised the concepts to make them make sense. Taking the concepts 'limited time' and 'numerous responsibilities' and putting them side by side and linking them to the concept 'health care professionals' with the linking word 'have' makes each proposition meaningful.

7   The inclusion of feelings: The inclusion of feelings will not be possible in all concept maps, but it is surprising how often including emotions and values related to the topic will change the meaning of the map. Refer to Figure 4.9.

How to use concept mapping for learning

1   Summaries of readings: As you read chapters, articles and websites you may find it useful to summarise your reading by constructing a concept map of the key concepts. Your maps can make an excellent summary of the subject's readings and you will probably find reviewing them very helpful when preparing for exams. Please note that it is possible to find that an author mentions concepts which are not then integrated with the material the chapter is discussing and so you may find it difficult to determine where these concepts 'fit in'. If you are having trouble fitting concepts into your map, you can always ask your teacher or other students for help.

2   A summary of the subject's work: As the subject progresses and your understanding of the topic develops you will be able to make more connections between concepts. You may find it useful to develop a 'high-level', overarching concept map of the entire subject. In a high-level map you will be looking to include the bigger concepts. Specific details and examples may not fit into a map that reflects the breadth of the entire subject. Such a map can help you to visualise how each of the bigger topics in the subject fit together.

3   Summaries of lecture notes: Concept mapping lecture notes helps students to summarise and understand lectures. At the end of the subject, studying one or two maps for each lecture is much easier than studying pages and pages of notes. At some stage you may even feel confident enough to construct maps during lectures.

4   Writing assignments: Students often have difficulty planning and sequencing the information they wish to present in an assignment. Mapping the assignment may assist you to sequence your material and produce a coherent, integrated assignment. We will discuss this further in Chapter 5.

Remember that the function of a concept map is to help [you to] structure [your] understanding of a topic and to create personal meaning. The value of concept mapping lies in [drawing the relationships and organising the hierarchy]. This process is not constrained to educational settings and so concept maps can be used in many different settings, [including work]. It can actually be used to help you to make sense of your world. And making sense of the world is no mean fcat!

(Fraser, 1996, p. 39)

The next chapter

Written assignments are a common form of assessment for health care courses. The following chapter discusses how to improve your academic writing. It goes through how to plan a writing timetable during the semester and focuses on the different elements of an assignment, addressing criteria. The chapter makes explicit the difference between a good and a poor grade.

5 Writing

Learning outcomes

By the end of this chapter readers are expected to be able to:

- have a strategy for relaxing before writing
- plan a writing schedule to allow time for someone else to read their first draft and for the rewriting of the first draft
- understand the importance of addressing the marking criteria for an assignment and answering the question posed, and
- have an understanding of what is expected in each of the different elements of an assignment.

Introduction

Virtually every accredited course requires that students write for assessment. Writing can help us to learn and through writing we can demonstrate what we have learnt. Academic writing has particular requirements and conventions and we can improve our academic writing over time. Over many years I have found that practice, feedback from others and my own reflection have helped to improve my writing, first as a student and then as an academic. I clearly remember my first university assignment. I received a pass for it. I had worked very hard on that first assignment and was convinced that if in the first year I could achieve only a pass for assignments, then I would fail in later years. I went to see my teacher to try to find out what I could do to improve my work. It was one of the best things that I ever did as a student. For my next assignment I received a distinction. Talking with the teacher really helped me to improve my writing. As an academic, I still ask for feedback on my writing. By the time you read this chapter, a colleague will have read it and provided me with advice on how to improve it. If you take nothing else away from this chapter, the two things that I would have you do are: 1) ask someone else to read and comment on your work and 2) think about their comments.

It's not easy to sit down and write an assignment, especially if you haven't written one in a long time. It's easy to feel anxious that we don't know anything about the topic, or how to start, or we worry about our spelling and grammar. It's important to recognise that having to write for assessment can be scary. It's also important to recognise that there are things to know about writing assignments and once we know those things we can improve our writing. We are going to discuss some of those strategies to improve our writing in this chapter. First though, I want to touch on overcoming fear.

Overcoming fear

Many students begin their study feeling afraid of writing for assessment. There are a couple of things that you can do to help allay those fears. First, deep breathing can help calm anxiety. One approach that I find helps to calm me down goes as follows: I close my mouth, breathe in through my nose for the count of four, hold my breath for the count of seven, and breathe out through my mouth for the count of seven. I repeat this sequence four more times. It's important for these breaths to be deep breaths that fill the lungs and move the diaphragm down. It is also helpful to do this half a dozen times during the day, not only when I am anxious.

Second, think about the writing that you currently do in your day-to-day personal and working life. What sorts of things do you write: lists, email messages, hand-over notes, memos at work, case notes, progress notes, condition reports and programme reports? The writing that you do for assessment may be a little more structured and specific, but you probably already practise many elements of writing that you need to do for an assignment. These elements may include collecting information and materials, sequencing what you will write, linking different sections together, making an argument, evaluating something and reflecting on what you have written.

The third thing that you can do to overcome fear of writing is to start writing. Write the first sentence. You can write it in pencil or on a computer. Ignore mistakes initially. *Do not* cross the sentence out. You are not writing a good draft; you are a long way from doing that. Truly, you can strive for perfecting and polishing later. It may help you to start writing if you talk into a tape recorder and then write from your recording. If you do this, keep in mind that our conversational language isn't the same as our written language so you will probably need to change what you write from your recording. However it can be a very useful strategy to start writing.

I can't stress strongly enough not to cross out what you initially write. If I crossed out every sentence that I didn't like when I first wrote it, I would never write anything. I find it really important just to get something onto the page. Often I have to resequence what I have written, write more to link different paragraphs together and I always have to rewrite, polish and rework what I have written. For me writing is a little like doing a jigsaw puzzle. It can seem impossible to do at first. Doing one small section of the puzzle then means that I can add to it and eventually I manage to complete the puzzle, or in this current case, this chapter!

Timing

Timing is everything when writing an assignment. Many students finish their assignment in the wee hours of the morning that the assignment is due. They only ever do one draft. As assignment writers we need to plan our time so that we can have enough time to ask someone to read our first draft and then rewrite our draft at least once.

To do this it will help to develop a writing plan. In week 2 of his first semester, Ben's class is given a 2000-word assignment which is due in week 10. The day that he was given the assignment Ben made a schedule for writing the assignment by the tenth week. He remembered writing high-school assignments the night before they were due. His marks were never very good and Ben wants to do well at university.

His schedule, which is shown in Table 5.1, shows that he will allow two weeks to gather the information and three weeks to write the first draft and find any further information needed. Ben plans on writing two drafts with over a week between the drafts. Two different people will read each draft. This may seem like a lot of time over which to write an assignment. However, during his undergraduate course Ben will need to write many assignments and he wants to learn as much as he can from writing his first few assignments so he will find it easier and perhaps quicker to write assignments in later semesters.

Table 5.1 A schedule or plan for writing Ben's 2000-word assignment

Week	Tuesday
2	Assignment given, develop timeline for writing, read three articles suggested.
3	Plan assignment headings, include relevant assessment criteria under relevant headings, check other sources of information (web, CINAHL database, etc.).
4	Write 1000 words (search for any more information needed). Talk with teacher if necessary.
5	Write the next 1000 words (search for any further information needed).
6	Draft the first version of the assignment. Remember transitions between sections.
7	Ask someone else to read the assignment (family member, friend, etc.).
8	Think about the feedback and write draft two.
9	Check reference list – make sure all references in the text match those in the reference list and all references in the list are in the text. Leave second draft for two days and then re-read and improve.
10	Assignment due, ask Anne to read three days before it is due and provide feedback. Night before the assignment is due, read for last time and submit.

Writing well can take time. You can expect to decrease the amount of time you need to write assignments during your course. You may also need to be strategic about your time because you may have other assignments to do for other subjects and you may not have as much time as you would like.

The structure of an assignment

There are many different types of assignments that you may be asked to write during your studies. While each assignment type has similarities (introduction, conclusion), the different types require you to demonstrate different outcomes. In Table 5.2 I have chosen to compare and contrast three typical assignments given in health care courses: the limited literature review, the research assignment and the case study. As you work your way through the table you will see that there is a typical structure for each type of assignment and you will see that many of the subheadings are the same. They all include a title or question and have an introduction in which you are expected to introduce to the reader what the assignment is about – the issue or problem to be explored and the significance or relevance of the problem. The three types of assignments require a literature review in which you demonstrate your knowledge of the key ideas that have been written about the topic. It's at this point that the assignment requirements begin to vary. In the literature review of the research assignment you will need to show how your research (the intervention or change that you will bring about) fits with what has already been written. This aspect is not required in the other two assignment types.

The research assignment also has a methodology and results section which the other two assignments don't have. In a research assignment you are expected to carry out an investigation. This might require laboratory work, a review of case notes, or an audit of an aspect of a clinical setting. In the methodology you need to give a very detailed account of what you did and how you did it so that another person can carry out your exact research and then confirm or refute your results. In the results section you are expected to display your results. You may find it useful to transform your results information into tables, figures, photographs and so on.

The case study has a section in which you are required to provide very specific details of the case. For instance, if your case study was of a particular patient, you may include personal information about the patient (age, gender, job, part of the country they live in, etc.). You may also need to include information about the health history of the person, the treatment they had received at different times and the outcomes of that treatment. You then use this very detailed information to show if the case study contradicts or supports the literature. You may also need to make recommendations about ways forward or further research.

All three of the assignment types will require you to write conclusions and have a reference section. You may also have appendices. If you do, you need to ensure that they are referred to in the text of your assignment.

Table 5.2 Structures of three different types of assignments

A literature review (this is a limited literature review, not a systematic literature review that you would find in the Cochrane database)	**A research assignment** (this is an assignment which often requires that the student carry out an intervention in order to change practice – e.g. review clinical practices and introduce a change to practice and compare outcomes)	**A case study** (this is an in-depth study of a single example of an issue, e.g. through a study of a patient, a clinic, a hospital department, a system, etc.)
Title/question – your literature review must relate to the actual or implicit question in the title	**Title/question** – your research assignment must address the actual or implicit question in the title. For a research assignment you may be required to state a hypothesis that your research then seeks to prove or disprove	**Title/question** – your case study must address the actual or implicit question in the title
Introduction – identifies the problem or the issue and perhaps justifies your choice of topic by discussing the significance of the problem	**Introduction** – discusses the problem, and perhaps justifies your choice of topic by discussing the significance of the problem	**Introduction** – discusses the problem and why the case study was undertaken. You may need to justify your choice of topic by discussing the significance of the problem
Literature review – demonstrates that you are aware of the important literature on this topic. It may be useful to structure this section by idea/concept/issue and report what the literature says about each	**Literature review** – demonstrates that you are aware of the important literature on this topic. Shows how your research fits with previous findings. It may be useful to structure this section by idea/concept/issue and report what the literature says about each	**Literature review and background** – this section introduces both the case itself and the literature which is relevant to the issues raised in the case study
	Methodology – detailed, step-by-step description of how you did your research and why you did what you did. Exact conditions, numbers of people interviewed/seeds planted, type of instruments used, etc. must be described	**The case** – detailed description of the case, for example a description of an intervention, the result of that intervention (in terms of the patient and other people), an evaluation of the intervention, issues or problems associated with the outcomes and their possible causes and solutions

Describe the audit or measurement criteria that you used. The methodology presents enough information so that someone else can exactly replicate your study. Some details (e.g. survey questions) may be best presented in an appendix and referred to in the methodology

Results – present your main findings using appropriate headings, tables, figures, etc. The text of your results section needs to refer to and make comment on any tables and figures

Discussion – This is the section where you analyse and explain your results. Explain if your results support your hypothesis or what you expected to find or not. In this section you are expected to make a comment on the reliability and validity of your results and explain any particular weaknesses in your methodology

Conclusions and recommendations – do not introduce any new material. Summarise your main arguments/themes and state your conclusions or recommendations. Explicitly link back or refer to your hypothesis/title. Support or reject if you have an hypothesis. Make clear why your conclusions are significant. Your recommendations may refer to further research or other ways to move forward

Conclusions and recommendations – this section is used to show if the case study contradicts or supports the literature. You may be asked to make recommendations about ways forward or further research. Try to refer explicitly back to the title or question in this section to demonstrate that your assignment has addressed the question asked

Discussion – in this section you critique the literature reviewed by evaluating the literature, comparing and contrasting (find similarities and differences), making comment on the significance of the literature, or stating an opinion. Whatever you do in the discussion you need to refer specifically to the literature that you reviewed. Don't introduce new literature in this section

Conclusions and recommendations – do not introduce any new material. Summarise your main arguments/themes and state your conclusions or recommendations. Explicitly link back or refer to the title. Make clear why your conclusions are significant. Your recommendations may refer to further research or other ways to move forward

Table 5.2 Structures of three different types of assignments *continued*

References – list all references used in your literature review. Double-check to make sure that you don't cite materials in your references that you haven't used in your review, and that all materials cited are in your references. Use the referencing style required	**References** – list all references used in your literature review. Double-check to make sure that you don't cite materials in your references that you haven't used in your assignment, and that all materials cited are in your references. Use the referencing style required	**References** – list all references used in your literature review. Double-check to make sure that you don't cite materials in your references that you haven't used in your case study, and that all materials cited are in your references. Use the referencing style required
Appendices – essential 'extra' information may be presented in appendices – e.g. a copy of national guidelines. Every appendix needs to be referred to in the text	**Appendices** – essential 'extra' information may be presented in appendices – e.g. a copy of survey questions. Every appendix needs to be referred to in the text	**Appendices** – essential 'extra' information may be presented in appendices – e.g. patient history details. Every appendix needs to be referred to in the text

Please note that the structures outlined in Table 5.2 are only to be used as guides. It is possible that your teacher will provide you with a slightly different structure for an assignment of the type demonstrated in the table and you will need to write according to the structure given.

One framework for writing an assignment

There are different ways to approach writing an assignment. Some students like to start writing. Some students prefer to make a list of all of the headings they expect to use in the assignment and then they write within each heading. Some students write paragraphs and pieces as they read for the assignment and then 'thread' the pieces together. For different assignments the same student may use different approaches. *There isn't one right way to go about writing an assignment.* Writing is a process that people make their own and refine over time. One of the great things about writing is that we all have the opportunity to experiment and work out for ourselves what we need to do to write well. Below I describe one way of going about the process of writing an assignment. You may find some or all of the elements of this approach to be useful.

Writing for a purpose

The teacher has asked you to write an assignment in order that you demonstrate your understanding of a topic. You need to be sure about what you have been asked to demonstrate. You may need to demonstrate your understanding of the literature, national guidelines and standards. You may need to critically review the literature. You may need to demonstrate that you can argue a case, compare and contrast different approaches or write guidelines. Are you asked to write for a particular audience – a patient group, manager or peers? It's essential that you determine the purpose of your assignment. Part of the purpose will be to write in a set number of words. It's important that you write within the word count. There are many different things that you could be asked to demonstrate through an assignment and you won't get any marks for doing something different, so you need to start by being sure you know what you are expected to achieve. The assignment criteria will help you and we will look more closely at criteria later in this chapter. Table 5.2, in which we compared the structure of a limited literature review, a research assignment and a case study, will also help you if your assignment is one of those types.

Answering the question

A common error that students make when writing assignments is that they don't actually answer the question or address the problem posed in the assignment. It is absolutely essential that you are clear about what the assignment requires you to do. If you have any doubts at all, talk with your teacher (or another student or colleague). You are not being stupid by talking with the teacher. You are being strategic; you are making sure you understand the teacher's intentions in setting the assignment.

Developing your ideas for the topic

As we discussed in Chapter 3 some teachers provide students with a degree of choice when setting assignments. You may have the opportunity to choose between topics, or choose a topic yourself. When you have this chance, it's useful to choose something that interests you or that you find motivating in some way. Perhaps you will be able to choose something that relates to the work that you do or uses information that you use at work. For example, you might be able to do an audit of some aspect of your practice. Doing an assignment that is related to your work or one that you have chosen yourself can help you to find both the time and the motivation to complete your assignment. If you have the opportunity to choose your own topic you need to make sure that:

- there is some literature on the topic to which you can refer
- your topic has a discrete focus. Students often choose topics that are too broad and so have problems completing the assignment, and
- there is something to debate/argue/review/find a gap in-between what is known and what needs to be known/make recommendations about as to a way forward/or make an improvement to, in your choice of topic.

If you are given the opportunity to choose your topic, it can be helpful to talk with your teacher or another student or a colleague about the topic you want to explore to make sure that you are on the right track. Also talk with the person about focusing the topic so that it is the right size, depth and word length.

Structuring

There is a proverb that suggests that it can be helpful to 'begin with the end in mind'. Thinking about the structure of the assignment before you start gathering further information and ideas and before you start writing may help you to see:

- which areas you still need to read about
- how all the pieces that you have been thinking and learning about may fit together
- what arguments you are going to need to make, and
- what you will need to do to 'link' all of the different sections of your assignment to make a coherent whole.

The structure of your assignment will depend on what you are asked to do. Table 5.2 provides examples of the structure for three different types of assignments. Your course may provide you with a structure to follow in your assignment, or the marking criteria may alert you to other headings that you will need to use.

Make a list of what you already know/have and what you need to do/find/read. Develop the headings and subheadings that you expect to use in your assignment. These headings are a starting place and unless prescribed, they aren't cast in stone. You can change them as you develop your first draft. Refer to Table 5.3 below. Marisa has been asked to do a project to improve an aspect of her clinic's practice. She has chosen to try to improve the glycaemic control of people with diabetes. The teacher provided the headings for the project and they are almost the same as for the research assignment in Table 5.2. However, instead of having a separate

Table 5.3 Marisa's research assignment. The headings were given as part of the marking criteria and having decided the topic (glycaemic control), Marisa has written down what she thinks she will need to collect/do for each heading. At this stage she doesn't have subheadings

Heading (given by the teacher)	Subheading (if relevant)	What I have/know	What I need to do
Introduction		Diabetes Control and Complication reference, National Service Framework.	Find another two references about glycaemic control, and GP contract incentives. Identify standards, compare with current practice.
Methodology		Determined criteria for choosing sample. Identified sample. Collected pre-intervention glycaemic control data.	Analyse patient cases, and determine post-intervention glycaemic control data. Develop intervention protocol, implement protocol, compare with previous glycaemic control data.
Results/ outcomes			Present pre and post data graphically if appropriate. Report protocol in appendix.
Discussion/ conclusions and recommendations			Compare pre and post data and discuss impact of protocol on patient glycaemic control, whole practice approach, management buy in. Refer to possible methodology weaknesses.
References			Make sure that each reference is in the text and is formatted.
Appendices			Refer to appendices in the text. Label appendices appropriately.

section for the literature review, the teacher asked for the literature to be reviewed in the introduction and she has asked for the discussion, conclusions and recommendations to sit within one section of the assignment. As you can see from Table 5.3, once she decided on the topic, Marisa was able to identify what she already knew/had, what information she still needed to look for, and what she had to do in each section to fulfil key marking criteria. For example, in the introduction Marisa has some of the relevant literature that she needs to refer to, but she needs to look for a couple more articles on glycaemic control and GP contract incentives and then do a comparision of the national standards with the current practice of the clinic.

Finding and recording information

Your teacher may have given you a full reading list or a few important readings that are keys to the topic. You may need to find further information for your assignment. Your sources of information might be DVDs, CD-ROMs, national guidelines, books, websites, blogs, articles, newspapers, surveys, reports, interviews, databases (refer to Chapter 2) or your own experience. Remember to seek the advice of the librarian, other students and colleagues. Keeping a notebook to record your ideas, information and references may be helpful. In reality you could spend all of your time finding information, opinions and arguments about the topic. However, you have to be selective. This is where your headings can help. As you read, collect information that you need for the headings you have already selected. Your reading may lead you to change your headings, add to them, or delete some (unless they are required by the marking criteria). Generally speaking, you need to focus your reading and information gathering. Your headings will help you to do this. Remember you have a word limit, so keep that in mind as you collect relevant information. Cottrell (2003, p. 152) suggests asking yourself two questions as you read:

1 Do I need the information?
2 How will I use this information?

Something that can waste a lot of time is taking poor notes on the sources of your information. Students forget to:

1   take down information about the book, journal, website (e.g. Fowler, J., Gudmundsson, A., and Whicker, L. (2006) *Groups Work*, Queensland: Australian Academic Press). Forgetting to take a note of the publisher or the place of publication means that your references aren't complete. It will take valuable time to go back and search for that reference.

2   note the page number for that quote – you found the perfect quote to introduce your argument, but you didn't note the page number. Again, it will take valuable time to find that information again.
3   show which of your notes are direct quotes or your interpretation of what you were reading. There are different ways that you can use to remind yourself which notes are direct quotes and which are your own words. Quotation marks (' '), italics and colour coding can help to identify direct quotes.

It's essential to be careful in the taking of your notes. You also need to be careful in the time you take reading for your assignment. Delineate a time-line, as Ben did in Table 5.1, so you know just how much time you can spend collecting your information and ideas before you need to start writing the assignment. Finding information and evidence to develop your assignment can be very time-consuming. Leaving it until the last minute to start your search is likely to influence negatively the quality of your assignment.

Writing

In Chapter 4 I discussed the use of concept mapping to pull together the key ideas in a topic and show explicitly how they are related. The technique can be used to help with the writing of an assignment. Concept mapping the topic of your assignment can help you to determine the sequence of head-ings in your assignment. A link from one concept to another can help you to write the transition sentence between one section and the next. If you are having a 'writing block', drawing a concept map can then help you to write from that map. For example, each link may be expanded to become a para-graph in your assignment. Mapping the assignment may also assist you to produce a coherent, integrated assignment.

First draft

When you are trying to write an assignment it's usual to write several drafts. In fact it's good practice to write several drafts. The first draft is 'seriously' a draft. All you are trying to do in the first draft is get down some of your ideas. You aren't trying to write the perfectly composed case study, essay or research assignment. Your ideas in the first draft may not be in the best order, the draft may have lots of spelling and grammatical errors, and the writing may not flow well. It's just a first draft and will need further work. The first draft is meant to have mistakes in it and it is meant not be fully thought out. In a later draft you can develop your ideas more, work on spelling, grammar and layout. In a later draft you will need to work on the transitions and flow. If you are having difficulty starting the first draft, let yourself start with whichever section feels the easiest to do. You don't always have to start at the beginning.

Second draft

In the second draft of your assignment you are working to ensure that you have demonstrated an understanding of the issues and complexities of the topic and made an argument (if appropriate) which is supported by the literature (i.e. references to relevant literature). You may need to show that you have evaluated the literature (made a judgement about the literature), or developed recommendations for change, again, based on the relevant literature. When you work on your second draft you need to check that you have answered the question or addressed the topic that was set. You will also need to:

- correct spelling and grammatical errors
- ensure that your writing flows and makes sense
- develop transitions between sections (this usually means writing a sentence or two at the end of one section that leads the reader into the following section – for example the last paragraph on the last page of Chapter 1 of this book is a transition to Chapter 2)
- make sure that all references in your assignment are in your reference list
- use examples and references that support your ideas, and
- correctly use the reference style required.

Ben

> At high school I was always losing marks for not using the correct referencing style, like Chicago or the American Psychological Association referencing style. Anne, my girlfriend said that I should use a programme like End Note so that I would get my references right. I went to an End Note lesson at the library and I am really pleased that I did. The programme has hundreds of different referencing styles and at the press of a button my references are correctly formatted for me. No more lost marks because I haven't got my references in the right style. The programme also requires that I put in all of the referencing information. I make a point of putting my references into the programme immediately I get them so I can make sure that I have all of the information that the programme needs.

The use of software like End Note is one way in which you can improve your references. A non-technical solution is to make a copy of examples of the referencing style your course requires and put them in your notebook. Any time that you read a journal article, website, book, conference poster or report that you may utilise in your assignments, write the reference down in your notebook and refer to the correct style as you enter the information. That way you can get the style right the first time you write the reference.

Polishing and finalising your assignment: asking someone to read it

You may never be satisfied with your assignment. You may feel that you could continue to make improvements to your assignment forever. However you will need to balance continuing to make changes with your need for time to work on other things and to submit the assignment on the due date. In the week before your assignment is due, final editing can take place. Make sure that you ask someone (partner, friend, work colleague, another student) to read your assignment. This is not cheating. You are not asking the person to write your assignment for you. You are asking them to proof-read it for you and tell you if it flows well, makes sense, and addresses the question/topic. The person doesn't have to know about the topic to do this. If they do know about the topic they may suggest other ideas about the content that you can consider. While it is important to consider their advice you don't have to take all advice given. It's your choice. Finally, in the week that the assignment is due, try to make sure that you leave a couple of days in which you don't look at your assignment so that you can read it one last time with 'fresh' eyes before submitting it.

Using teacher feedback on your assignment

When assignments are returned many students look only at the grade. Often a grade doesn't tell you how to improve your work for future assignments. It is incredibly valuable to take the time to reread your assignment in light of the comments made by the teacher. If you don't understand the comments, or can't see how to improve from the feedback, I strongly urge you to talk with the teacher about improving your work. The vast majority of teachers really want to help their students to improve their work and will take the time to help you to do this.

Addressing the criteria

Laboratory reports, projects, essays and case studies, are all different types of 'assignments'; however they do have elements in common. All are written, all require a logical structure, transitions and clarity of expression, and all have *criteria* against which your work will be assessed. While I won't discuss each of these types of written assignments, I am going to discuss the addressing of the specific criteria for a specific research assignment. The ideas about addressing criteria can be transferred equally well to the writing of other types of assignments.

I am indebted to Anne McDermott who from 2004 to 2007 was the Course Director for the Warwick Diabetes Care Certificate in Diabetes Care (University of Warwick). Anne very kindly gave me permission to use the criteria and guidelines that Warwick Diabetes Care developed for the student research assignment used in its certificate. I have modified the criteria and guidelines for the purposes of this chapter.

Criteria for a research assignment

Below I discuss each of the criteria that the Certificate in Diabetes Care used for the elements of the research assignment that students of the course are asked to produce. Students are required to carry out a piece of research and write their assignment using the following headings: Introduction, Methodology, Results, Discussion, References and Appendices. There is also a criterion for presentation of the project and a 3000-word limit. For this piece of assessment, students are asked to conduct a piece of research to improve the practice of diabetes care in their workplace. While Marisa chose to look at improving glycaemic control for a specific subset of clinic patients, many different areas could be chosen, for example, retinopathy screening, patient education or changes to clinic documentation/protocols.

Introduction

The criteria for the introduction of this assignment are:

- states the aim of the assignment
- contains sufficient depth and breadth of the chosen topic area
- includes key references for the topic area
- shows the significance of the topic.

The introduction gives the reader (and the marker) a clear idea of what you hope to achieve in the assignment (the aim) and why you are doing it. There needs to be enough information so that what you are doing makes sense to the reader. To demonstrate the significance of the topic in the introduction, Marisa, who is working on glycaemic control, would show that specific literature says that glycaemic control reduces microvascular complications. This demonstrates to the marker that she has good reasons for her choice of topic. The introduction needs to refer to *relevant* evidence. The references need to be related to the topic and must be cited correctly. Remember, a long list of references not really related to the topic will not enhance the assignment.

Methodology

The criteria for the methodology are:

- related to the aim
- reproducible.

The methodology should describe clearly and in depth what process you have gone through to complete the research. Think about 'what, when, where, who, how and why'. What did you do, when did you do it, where did you do it, who did you do it to, how did you do it and why did you decide to do it that way? It needs to be clear enough to enable someone else to follow your method. Assume the reader knows nothing about what you do. So, for example if the research was about patient education sessions, you would need to include:

- what you did to set them up, including whether you had any meetings, did literature searches, etc.
- when you will deliver them, or propose to deliver them, if the project is preliminary work
- who your audience will be (not their names but the criteria used for selecting people)
- how you plan to deliver them, including whether questionnaires are to be designed or used, and
- why you decided on this type of approach.

The methodology provides as much detail as needed by someone else who wanted to repeat your work. This means that your work is reproducible.

The criteria also require the methods to be related to the project aim. For example, the aim of Marisa's project is to try to improve patient glycaemic control through a particular intervention. As part of her methodology she searches her workplace computer-based records for patients with a HB^{a1c} of between 7.5 and 7.9. She links this part of the process to her aim with a sentence: 'In order to trial the intervention which is the aim of this project, I needed first to select a sample of patients who had poor glycaemic control. I also needed to limit the number of people in this trial and so I chose patients with a HB^{a1c} of between 7.5 and 7.9.'

Results

The criteria for the results are:

- related to the methodology
- includes final or interim results/outcomes.

The results need to show what you have produced from your research. The results could be resources produced, policies and procedures changed or produced, data from questionnaires or biochemistry, changes in knowledge and attitudes, etc. The text should include summaries of any results (for instance in tables or graphs) and the full results placed in the appendices if too long for the assignment text. It's important that any appendices are referred to in the text of the assignment. Any tables, figures and graphs need to be referred to appropriately. Do not assume the reader will automatically understand your tables or figures. You will need to explain the key elements about your tables and figures in the text. Any sources of diagrams used need to be acknowledged. The results should show the outcomes of the work you did (your methodology).

In order to show that your results are linked to your methodology you need to show the reader that each set of results comes from the work that you did. For example, Marisa might show the relationship by writing in her results section 'The before and after intervention HB^{a1c} results that were collected are illustrated in Table 1'. The use of very specific subheadings may be another way to show the relationship. The results can't include data from anywhere other than the work that you did. For example, they can't be from a published piece of research or a national framework.

Discussion

The criteria for the discussion are:

- reflects on the strength/weakness of your methods
- reflects on the strength/weakness of your results
- reflects on the effect on clinical practice
- reflects on results compared with the evidence base.

The discussion allows you to take a step back and comment on your work. Look at what you have produced and critically appraise it. Has it been successful? Were the results as you would have expected? Could the work that you did be adapted? What could you have done differently with hindsight? It may be appropriate to compare your results with both local and national guidelines. Link this section to the introduction evidence base as much as possible, e.g. 'Out of a group of twenty invited people with diabetes, there were fifteen who attended all the sessions and 20 who attended at least three out of the four planned sessions. This was a similar finding to ... (reference)'.

References

The criteria for the references are:

- cited adequately in the text and in the reference list
- has at least ten references.

For these criteria you need to include a minimum of ten relevant references. Every reference in your reference list needs also to be found in the text of your assignment and vice versa. This is something that a friend could check for you. You must not put references in that you have not used in the text of your assignment. The text should be referenced appropriately and the reference list included after the discussion and before the appendices. References should be cited using the referencing style your teacher has asked you to use (e.g. Harvard, Chicago). Remember, you can use a range of references such as websites, newspaper articles, journal articles, reports, conference papers and so on. Only use one referencing style.

Appendices

The criteria for the appendices are:

- present, labelled and referred to in the text
- contain factually correct and up-to-date information.

Include all of the material that supports your assessment, but which does not have a place within the main body of text. Appendices should be relevant and correct and referred to in the text of the project.

Presentation

Often assignments, laboratory reports, etc. also include a criterion about the presentation of the work for which marks will be awarded. This generally isn't about the quality of the cover into which you put your assignment. It's more about the ease of reading your project (font size and margins so that there is enough white space for the marker), spelling and grammatical errors (can be improved by having a friend read your assignment), and whether the assignment is clear, logical and understandable.

The difference between a good and a poor grade

I am indebted to Professor Sandra Dunn from Charles Darwin University for allowing me to use the grading system guidelines that the School of Graduate Health Practice uses in its assessment of written work. I have slightly modified the guidelines for the purposes of this chapter (Tables 5.4 and 5.5). As you will see from Table 5.4, the School of Graduate Health Practice at Charles Darwin University grades students using five categories ranging from a 'high distinction' to a 'fail'. Each grade is described in the table. You can see from the table that as the grades increase the student is expected to demonstrate a more sophisticated understanding of the subject.

Table 5.5 provides the criteria used to assess assignments in the School of Graduate Health Practice and gives a detailed description of the requirements for each criterion from a high distinction to a fail. The description for each individual criterion is aligned to the overall description of the grade found in Table 5.4. Let's compare the achievement required of one criterion. You can then look across the range of grades for the other criteria to help

Table 5.4 An example grading system

Grade	Description	Percentage
High distinction (HD)	Demonstrates imagination, originality or flair, based on proficiency in all learning outcomes of the subject; work is interesting or surprisingly exciting, challenging, well read or scholarly	85–100
Distinction (D)	Demonstrates awareness and understanding of deeper and less obvious aspects of the subject, such as ability to identify and debate critical issues or problems, ability to solve non-routine problems, ability to adapt and apply ideas to new situations, and ability to evaluate new ideas	75–84
Credit (C)	Demonstrates ability to use and apply fundamental concepts and skills of the subject, going beyond mere replication of content knowledge or skill to show understanding of key ideas, awareness of their relevance, some use of analytical skills, and some originality or insight	60–74
Pass (P)	Satisfies all of the basic learning requirements of the subject, such as knowledge of fundamental concepts and performance of basic skills; demonstrates satisfactory, adequate, competent, or capable achievement of the learning outcomes for the assignment	50–59
Fail (F)	Does not satisfy the basic learning outcomes for the assignment	0–49

you to understand what assessors are looking for when they grade your written work.

If we compare the grades for the criterion 'concepts and theories' we will see that the assessor is looking for four different elements to grade the paper: understanding of concepts, analysis, relevance of material used, and answering the question (Table 5.6). The first two elements in particular are used to distinguish between all of the grades. To be at the level of high distinction in this criterion you need to be able to demonstrate to the assessor that you have really understood the relevant literature and that you have analysed the ideas presented and made a critical comment about the literature. A lower level of grade on this criterion means that you haven't demonstrated an in-depth understanding of the literature, analysed the literature, reflected upon it and made critical comment. The assessment of citing relevant materials and answering all aspects of the question also contribute to the grade for this criterion.

Table 5.5 provides an example of a grading scheme for written assessment. Your course may also provide a grading scheme, but if it doesn't, then this example will give you an idea of the sorts of aspects that your assessor may be looking for to grade your work. Your teacher may also provide examples of assignments that were given different grades. If so, take the

Table 5.5 Assignment grading guideline matrix

Criteria	High distinction	Distinction	Credit	Pass	Fail
Introduction (5%) Paper provides a clear introduction	Introduction offers clear outline of paper and provides direction for the discussion	Introduction offers clear outline of paper and provides direction for the discussion	Introduction offers outline of paper or provides direction for the discussion	Introduction attempts to offer outline of paper or provide direction for the discussion	Limited or no introduction
Literature (20%) Demonstrated use of relevant literature	Literature cited is relevant and extensive; consistent evidence of wide reading	Literature cited is relevant; some evidence of wide reading	Literature cited is appropriate and covers all crucial points; readings limited to study materials	Some literature cited; only some references relevant to argument	Limited or no literature cited
Concepts and theories (25%) Demonstrated understanding of the topic and the concepts and theories used	Evidence of high level of understanding of concepts/theories used, demonstrates analysis, reflective and critical thinking; paper addresses all aspects of the question in an integrated way and contains no irrelevant material or repetition of ideas	Evidence of substantial understanding of concept/theories used, demonstrates some analysis, reflective and/or critical thinking; paper addresses all aspects of the question, includes no irrelevant material or repetition but has some weak connections between ideas	Partial understanding of concepts and theories, awareness of their relevance; attempt at analysis of issues; paper addresses only some aspects of the question and/or contains some irrelevant material and/or repetition of ideas	Evidence of understanding of fundamental concepts; some understanding of concepts/theories used; paper addresses only some aspects of the question and contains either irrelevant material or repetition of ideas	Limited or no understanding demonstrated; irrelevant materials used; repetition of ideas; paper does not answer the question

Table 5.5 Grading guideline matrix *continued*

	Criteria	High distinction	Distinction	Credit	Pass	Fail
Arguments and analysis (30%)	Coherent argument which is sustained by logic and evidence	Coherent and logical argument, extensively sustained by readings and evidence; argument reflects student's critical thinking and synthesis; argument demonstrates imagination, originality or flair	Well organised and clear argument sustained by readings and evidence; argument reflects student's critical thinking and synthesis of deeper and less obvious aspects of the argument; demonstrates ability to adapt and apply ideas to new situations	Some evidence of an argument with some support from readings and evidence, but is unclear in some important areas; shows some use of analytical skills, and some originality or insight	Mostly description rather than argument or the argument is not well supported, unclear or logically flawed with limited support	Limited or no argument, only description or personal opinion, with no supporting logic or evidence, isolated statements are made but are not connected in any logical way
Conclusion (10%)	Paper offers a purposive conclusion	Conclusion presents no new material; offers a summation of ideas, draws together the discussion and offers the student's 'position' drawn from the discussion in the body	Conclusion presents no new material; offers a summation of ideas, draws together the discussion and/or offers the student's 'position' drawn from the discussion in the body	Conclusion attempts to summarise the ideas or discussion, draws together the discussion or offers the student's 'position'drawn from the discussion in the body	Conclusion attempts to summarise the ideas or discussion; may offer the student's 'position'; limited linking to discussion	Limited or no conclusion

Criteria					
Writing style (5%)	Paper is written in formal academic style with clarity and coherence	High level of clarity in articulating and presenting issues and ideas in a concise, coherent manner	High level of clarity in articulating and presenting issues and ideas in a concise, coherent manner	Writing style is satisfactory and clear	Writing style is satisfactory and clear
Presentation (5%)	Paper meets referencing and presentation requirements for formal written work	Grammar, syntax, spelling, sentence and paragraph structure, paragraph linking, use of section headings are appropriate; accurate and systematic referencing; word count adhered to	Grammar, syntax, spelling, sentence and paragraph structure, paragraph linking, use of section headings are appropriate; accurate and systematic referencing	Paper contains occasional grammatical or spelling errors; inconsistent referencing; word count adhered to	Paper contains several grammatical or spelling errors, inappropriate language, and/or layout; inconsistent and/or incorrect referencing; word count not adhered to
Timeliness	Paper submitted when due or with approved extension				

Additional column (right):

Writing style is difficult to follow
Paper contains frequent grammatical or spelling errors, inappropriate language and layout; limited or no referencing; word count not adhered to

Table 5.6 Comparing grades for the criterion 'concepts and theories'

Elements of the criterion	High distinction	Distinction	Credit	Pass	Fail
Under-standing of concepts	High level of under-standing	Substantial under-standing	Under-standing of basic ideas and key ideas	Under-standing of basic ideas	No under-standing
Analysis/ critical thinking/ reflection	Demon-strated	Some demon-stration	Analysis attempted	No analysis	No analysis
Relevant material	No irrelevant material used, no irrelevant repetition of ideas, all ideas strongly connected	No irrelevant material used, no irrelevant repetition of ideas, some ideas only weakly connected	Some irrelevant materials used and/or some repetition of ideas	Some irrelevant materials used and/or some repetition of ideas	Irrelevant materials used, repetition of ideas
Answered the question	All aspects of question answered	All aspects of question answered	Some aspects of question answered	Some aspects of question answered	Question not answered

time, perhaps with another student, to read and analyse the assignments to determine the differences between them. If not, you may be able to:

- discuss your rough draft with your teacher
- ask another student who received a better grade for an assignment to share their paper with you and compare it with yours, or
- discuss your assessed paper with your teacher.

Improving your academic writing takes time, feedback and determination. Don't give in if your first assignment doesn't receive the grade you would have liked. Keep going and you will improve over time if you try even some of the ideas discussed so far in this chapter.

Plagiarism

I want to finish this chapter with a discussion of plagiarism because plagiarising has serious consequences for students and academics alike. If an academic plagiarises the work of another, they can lose their job. If a student plagiarises the work of another, they can fail the subject and even be expelled from the course. So what is plagiarism and how can we make sure we don't plagiarise?

Plagiarism, the appropriation or imitation of another's ideas and manner of expressing them, as in art, literature, etc. to be passed off as one's own.

(*Macquarie Dictionary*, 1991)

Studies in health care inevitably require us to be familiar with an evidence base. We are expected to know what the research literature and national guidelines say about the topics we're studying. We may also refer to topic discussions on the web, in newspapers, from interviews and via email discussion groups. When our assessment involves written work, we need to make sure that we appropriately quote and cite words, ideas and images that aren't our own. We need to give credit to others where it is due. Therefore a student must not intentionally or unintentionally:

• copy or buy someone else's assignment and pretend that it is theirs
• have a friend write an assignment for them and pretend that it is theirs
• reproduce someone else's words without using quotation marks and citing them regardless of whether their words were in an email, a book, journal article, on the web, etc. (e.g. 'Ramsden, 2003, p. 65')
• use someone else's ideas without citing them (citing refers to naming the author who wrote about the ideas – e.g. 'Fowler *et al.*, 2006')
• use someone else's images (charts, diagrams, illustrations, pictures, etc.) without citing them and showing the page number, and
• use their own previously published work without quoting it. In Chapter 4 I have used work that I have previously published and I had to quote that work (including page numbers) so as not to plagiarise my own work.

In our written work, citing others builds our credibility. It shows that we are familiar with the relevant literature. However our teachers generally expect us to show that we can build on the ideas of others with our own ideas; we need to show that we can evaluate, synthesise and analyse the ideas of others. So in our written work, we must be careful to distinguish clearly between what is ours and what is the work of others. It is important for your own integrity that there can be no possibility for misunderstanding in this area.

Distinguishing between the work of others and our own work takes time, effort and care. When we take notes we need always to use quotation marks when we copy words and images directly (and write down the reference and page number).

Sometimes students try to paraphrase some text. This means that they try to restate the meaning of the text in their own words. The following are examples of acceptable and unacceptable paraphrasing. I have quoted these examples directly from the Read Write Think professional development website which is a partnership between the United States of America-based

National Council of Teachers of English, the International Reading Association (IRA), and the MarcoPolo Education Foundation: http://www.readwritethink.org/lesson_images/lesson158/plagiarismactivity. pdf. The book being referenced is Williams *et al.* (1980).

HOW TO RECOGNIZE UNACCEPTABLE AND ACCEPTABLE PARAPHRASES

Here's the ORIGINAL text, from page 1 of *Lizzie Borden: A Case Book of Family and Crime in the 1890s* by Joyce Williams *et al.*:

> The rise of industry, the growth of cities, and the expansion of the population were the three great developments of late nineteenth century American history. As new, larger, steam-powered factories became a feature of the American landscape in the East, they transformed farm hands into industrial laborers, and provided jobs for a rising tide of immigrants. With industry came urbanization, the growth of large cities (like Fall River, Massachusetts, where the Bordens lived), which became the centers of production as well as of commerce and trade.

Here's an UNACCEPTABLE paraphrase that is **plagiarism**:

> The increase of industry, the growth of cities, and the explosion of the population were three large factors of nineteenth century America. As steam-driven companies became more visible in the eastern part of the country, they changed farm hands into factory workers and provided jobs for the large wave of immigrants. With industry came the growth of large cities like Fall River where the Bordens lived which turned into centers of commerce and trade as well as production.

WHAT MAKES THIS PASSAGE PLAGIARISM?
The preceding passage is considered plagiarism for two reasons:

- the writer has only changed around a few words and phrases, or changed the order of the original's sentences.
- the writer has failed to cite a source for any of the ideas or facts.

If you do either or both of these things, you are plagiarizing. **NOTE:** This paragraph is also problematic because it changes the sense of several sentences (for example, "steam-driven companies" in sentence two misses the original's emphasis on factories).

Here's an ACCEPTABLE paraphrase:

> Fall River, where the Borden family lived, was typical of northeastern industrial cities of the nineteenth century. Steam-powered production had shifted labor from agriculture to manufacturing,

and as immigrants arrived in the US, they found work in these new factories. As a result, populations grew, and large urban areas arose. Fall River was one of these manufacturing and commercial centers (Williams 1).

WHY IS THIS PASSAGE ACCEPTABLE?
This is acceptable paraphrasing because the writer:

- accurately relays the information in the original.
- uses her own words.
- lets her reader know the source of her information.

(Read Write Think, 2008)

Further examples of unacceptable paraphrasing can be found at the Indiana University Writing Tutorial Services web page: http://www.indiana.edu/~wts/pamphlets/plagiarism.shtml. The Georgetown University Academic Resource Center website provides tips about plagiarism at http://ldss.georgetown.edu/acad-plagiarism.cfm, and the Purdue University website 'Avoiding plagiarism': http://owl.english.purdue.edu/owl/resource/589/01/.

Tips

1   Pay attention to what you are asked to do – e.g. answer the question, use the section headings required, address the selection criteria, etc.
2   Finish your first draft so that you can leave it for a day and then reread it yourself/ask someone to read your draft. Pay attention to the comments you receive on your draft but don't feel obliged to accept all comments.

The next chapter

Assignments can be developed over a period of time. They can be reviewed and revised and feedback from others can be sought before submission. Students may also be asked to demonstrate their understanding in a shorter, more intense period of time through an exam. Some students believe they perform well under exam conditions while other students believe they don't. In the next chapter I discuss ways in which you can prepare for an exam and strategies that you can use in the exam itself to maximise your marks.

6 Preparing for and taking exams

Learning outcomes

By the end of this chapter readers are expected to be able to:

- choose how prepared you want to be for an exam
- plan the timing for answering exam questions at the beginning of the exam
- identify several strategies for choosing the correct answer in multiple-choice questions, and
- identify strategies for preparing for exam essay questions.

Introduction

Many subjects no longer include exams as part of the assessment. Academics increasingly value what is referred to as 'authentic assessment' which more closely reflects the situations in which we find ourselves in workplaces. Having said that, exams are still used in many courses. Exams allow us as students to show what we know and understand about the topics we have studied. While it is possible for a student to submit an assignment which s/he hasn't written, exams are organised such that it's likely that the exam answers are the student's own work. Almost all exams are invigilated (supervised) and if the invigilator doesn't know the students, students will be asked to show photo identification to prove their identity.

If you are particularly worried about taking exams, look for a course that doesn't use them as part of the assessment. If the course you are taking has exams and you are particularly worried – don't panic – there are ways to improve your preparation for and your taking of exams.

Preparation

Preparation for exams consists of several parts including:

- coping with stress

- choosing your level of preparation
- revising and refining notes
- practising with past exam papers, and
- the approach used on the exam day.

Coping with stress

A certain level of stress can be productive, helping us to operate at our peak. Too much stress, though, can hinder our performance and this is true of many things in life, not just study and taking exams. Personally, I find being well prepared helps me with my stress levels; however there are always times when I am not as well prepared as I would like to be. Exercise (even five or ten minutes walking up and down stairs) and deep breathing (as discussed in Chapter 5) help me to manage my stress levels. I also find the exercise of clenching specific muscles (fingers, toes, shoulders, etc.) and then releasing them to be helpful. Adequate sleep, good nutrition and a positive attitude (telling yourself that you can succeed) all help to reduce stress levels. An internet search will reveal many different sites with tips about how to manage stress.

Some students feel nervous and even panicked when they try to study. If this is the case for you, as well as using relaxation strategies, it may be useful for you to break your revision down into small, achievable pieces: 'I will spend the next half an hour finding all of my notes on topic X.' Doing so helps you to know the extent of your notes and having that overview will help you to plan your approach to summarising that topic. There are other strategies for helping yourself to start your revision, such as revising with another student and choosing to answer just one question from a past exam. Even if you don't know the answer, working through your notes or text to find the answer is part of your revision. If you find starting your revision difficult, choose small, achievable steps.

Choosing your level of preparation: it is your choice

Ideally for every exam we would prepare and revise gradually throughout the semester such that we are 100 per cent prepared by the day of the exam. Real life is not always like that so it is up to you to choose strategically the level of preparation for each exam. You don't have to be 100 per cent prepared for every exam. When you choose how prepared you would like to be, it's useful to take into consideration the value of the exam, whether you will pass the subject even if you fail the exam, how many exams you have to take, and whether you will have learnt what you want to learn even if you fail the exam.

For example, Ben is studying four subjects and is in his second semester of the first year of his three-year degree. In one subject the assessment includes two 40 per cent assignments and an end of subject 20 per cent exam. The subject does not require that each assessment element has to be passed in order to pass the subject. Ben has decided to put his time and focus for this subject into the assignments. He has done very well on his assignments in the first semester so he is confident that he can pass the subject through his assignments. Ben doesn't have any other end-of-semester exams so he is going to focus on revising for this one exam in the study week before the exam. He knows that cramming isn't the best way to prepare. He believes that in that week he will be able to cover seven of the thirteen topics that the exam may cover. Ben has made a strategic choice about how best to use his limited time. He might well have made a very different choice if the exam was worth 50 per cent or more or if he needed to pass all assessments in order to pass the subject.

Revising and refining notes

Cramming just prior to the exam rarely produces the exam results we would like. Ideally, revision of topics starts early in the semester and continues in a measured way up until the exam. Some students dedicate their holidays and long weekends to their revision schedule. It may not be practical for you to review all of your topics and review all of the material that was covered and allocated during the semester. Again we need to be strategic in our revision planning. Looking at the learning outcomes and past exam questions will help you to focus your revision. It's likely to be useful for you to review your assignments, lecture notes and chapter notes. Distilling new, summarising notes from your subject materials will help you to focus on the key aspects of the subject.

Table 2.3 illustrates a semester-long revision plan based on the number of topics and doing two past exam papers. Kris from Table 2.3 is studying a module which has a 60 per cent end-of-semester exam. She has decided to revise all of the way through the semester. There are five broad topic areas studied in the module and her aim is to distil all of her notes from lectures, chapter and journal article reading, and the online discussions into two to three concept maps for each topic. Kris has lots of notes from each week of her module. She wants to pull together the key ideas, facts and concepts from each of those weeks into a manageable form. When it comes to the last few days before the exam, she wants to be able to study a dozen or so concept maps that summarise all of the topics in the subject. Kris is also going to prepare one page of 'facts' that she feels she needs to memorise for this module. To summarise the semester she will need to choose the key ideas or concepts in each of the topics. She is guided by the learning outcomes for each topic area, past exam papers and her own understanding of the topics. Kris could choose to try to summarise the topics through notes rather than concept maps. To do this she could try to limit her notes to two or three pages for each topic area. To do this she will still need to distil the key ideas of each topic.

One strategy that can be very useful in helping to make summarising notes or concept maps is to identify several key questions (and their answers) that reflect what the topic is all about. What question would you ask to capture the key concepts in this topic? If you don't have a text that already provides questions or your teacher hasn't done this, it may be very helpful for you or you and a group of other students to try to do this for yourselves.

Once you have distilled your summary notes it will be helpful to reread them two or three times in the couple of days just prior to the exam. Please don't try to memorise all of your notes. There will be elements of your notes that you will probably need to memorise; for example you may need to remember formulae, or steps in a process. Make a separate list of the things that you do need to memorise. Some students also try to memorise the major headings of their summary notes. Knowing the headings reminds them of the key ideas about that topic, which can in turn remind them of the rest of the content.

Similarly there's not much point in trying to learn your summaries or essays off by heart. While it will be helpful to read them, you are probably wiser spending time doing practice exam questions and discussing exam questions with others rather than continually rereading your notes and essays.

Practising past exam papers

Past exam papers provide us with a lot of information and it is decidedly important that you do any past exam papers that you can. They won't necessarily tell you the actual questions that you will need to answer but they will let you know:

- the type of questions that you might be asked (factual recall, analysis, synthesis, etc.)
- the level of detail or understanding required by the questions (do you need to memorise a lot of information or understand the topic fully and in depth?)
- about the coverage of the exam (e.g. were all major topics covered or only some?)
- how individual learning outcomes for the module are assessed through an exam, and
- how to plan how much time to spend on each part of the exam.

Trying to answer the questions may also provide you with information about the areas that you may not know well enough yet. Practising past exam papers can help to focus your preparation further. I will touch on doing past exam papers again in the section on 'Types of exam questions'.

The approach used on the exam day

On the day of the exam itself we need to avoid added stress. Make sure that you arrive at the exam room with plenty of time to spare (at least ten minutes). This may mean that you need to ensure that you get up in time (set an alarm or have someone call you). In a large organisation such as a university it is likely that your exam will be held in a place that you haven't been to before. It will be useful to go there prior to the exam day so that you know exactly how to get to your exam room. You don't need the stress of not being able to locate the exact room on the day. Being late for an exam is never helpful for your state of mind.

Check beforehand to see what you may take into the exam. While you may be allowed to take in a calculator, ruler, pens, pencils, etc. you may find it helpful to have water, sweets or a snack.

In the exam itself there are certain requirements that you will need to abide by and strategies that you may find useful. The requirements will be things like 'do not open the exam paper before you are asked to do so' and 'do not talk with anyone except the invigilator during the exam'. The strategies that are important are related to pacing yourself and answering as many questions as you can so that you have the best chance of maximising your marks. For example:

- Often exams are organised such that you are allowed to read the exam paper before you can start writing. Doing so allows you to check things such as 'do I have the right exam and all of the questions/pages?' Make sure always to look at the back page to see if there are any questions there. A preliminary reading of the exam paper will also allow you to identify which questions you can do most easily. Start by doing those questions that you find the easiest as this will help you to feel more confident. It may be sensible to leave the questions that you find difficult to the end. By answering the questions that you find easiest you may also help yourself to maximise your marks.
- Pacing yourself so that you finish answering all questions will help you to maximise your marks. At the beginning of an exam it is worth taking a few minutes to decide how much time you will spend on each section. Questions may be weighted differently and this will need to be taken into consideration when allocating how much time you will spend on each question. Below are three different examples of allocating time during an exam.

  Example 1   To complete an eighty-question multiple-choice question (MCQ) exam in an hour you will need to answer twenty questions every fifteen minutes (this assumes that every question is worth the same number of marks). Keeping an eye on timing during the exam will help you not to spend too long on a few questions at the expense of not finishing the test. For example, if you were to spend fifteen minutes on four or five questions that you found difficult, you might not be able to finish the test and so potentially miss out on marks from answering questions that you would get right.

Example 2 Some short-answer and essay exams may have questions that are weighted differently. In a two-hour exam you may need to write two essays for 30 marks each, and answer ten short-answer questions for 40 marks. Dividing your time according to the number of marks will mean that you have approximately 36 minutes to write each essay and 48 minutes to answer the short-answer questions (or just under five minutes for each short-answer question). If you spend more time on your essays, say 45 minutes on each essay, while you might gain a few more marks on each essay, you then might not be able to finish each of the short-answer questions. If you couldn't finish four of the short-answer questions (because you had used 18 minutes extra on your essays) you would automatically lose 16 marks. It's not likely that the extra time spent on your essays would give you 16 more marks to make up for the marks lost through not doing the short-answer questions.

Example 3 A one-hour exam has one question of multiple parts that is worth half of the marks, while another nine questions comprise the other half of the marks. It would be sensible to allocate about half an hour to the first question and about three minutes to each of the other nine questions. It is worth a few minutes of your time at the beginning of the exam to calculate how long you can spend on each question. Again, start with the easiest questions to help calm your nerves and boost your confidence.

Table 6.1 shows an example of Kris's plan for how to allocate time during a two-hour-and-fifteen-minute exam, of which ten minutes is given to reading the exam before starting to write answers. During the two hours she is expected to answer eighty MCQs worth 80 marks, one essay worth 40 marks and five short-answer questions worth 40 marks (8 marks each). Kris has allocated two hours to do the exam, five minutes at the end to review, and ten minutes for the preliminary reading. One hour will be spent on the MCQs (80 marks) and the second hour on the essay and short-answer questions. She has split the first sixty minutes into four fifteen-minute blocks, in each of which she will try to answer 20 questions. In the second sixty-minute period she has allocated half an hour for the essay (40 marks) and half an hour (six minutes each) for the five short-answer questions (8 marks each). Kris has made a decision that she is likely to get more marks from the MCQ

Table 6.1 A plan for taking a two-hour-and-fifteen-minute exam with eighty MCQs worth 1 mark each, one essay worth 40 marks and five short-answer questions worth 40 marks. The first ten minutes are for reading only.

10.00–10.10	Fill out your name, student ID etc. on the exam answer sheets. Determine number of questions and plan time to allow for each section. Skim exam questions and decide what to start first.
10.10–10.25	Complete first 20 MCQs
10.25–10.40	Complete next 20 MCQs
10.40–10.55	Complete third set of 20 MCQs
10.55–11.10	Complete last set of 20 MCQs
11.10–11.16	Answer first short-answer question
11.16–11.22	Answer second short-answer question
11.22–11.28	Answer third short-answer question
11.28–11.34	Answer fourth short-answer question
11.34–11.40	Answer fifth short-answer question
11.40–11.45	Plan essay structure
11.45–12.10	Write essay
12.10–12.15	Check any questions that you need to return to. If you work through your questions more quickly than your plan, use the extra time to double-check any answers you aren't sure of or questions you haven't been able to answer

and short-answer questions so she is going to do those first. If she runs out of time she plans to make quick notes to answer the essay question. If she has extra time, she will be able to use it to finish the essay and check her other answers. Kris may not be able to stick exactly to the plan. What is important is that she has one. As she progresses through the exam Kris will try to stick with her plan but she may need to modify it slightly.

Types of exam question

Essays

Exam essays will need the same sort of approach that you use when writing essays that aren't written under exam conditions. Aspects that are important to the successful answering of exam essays include:

* answering the question
* having an argument/comparison/evaluation
* structuring the essay in a way that is logical and can be followed, and
* including any evidence that you have.

Remember to have an introduction and a conclusion that links back to the question that you were asked. Your exam essays will need to have easily identified sections and paragraphs, sentences that are well constructed and, if relevant, diagrams that are correctly labelled and appropriately referred to in the text of the essay.

Some students allocate several minutes to plan the outlines of their essays before starting to write their answers. Doing so helps them with the structure of their essays. Other students prefer to start writing immediately and structure as they go. There isn't one right way and you will need to work out what works best for you.

It's important not to try to include everything you know about the topic. You will have been asked to answer a specific question or look at a particular perspective. Including extraneous information, even if it is correct, won't win you extra marks. If you find that while working on your essay you are running out of time, at least jot down the main points that you were going to make, even if in bullet point form. Doing so may secure you some further marks.

When preparing for an essay exam it is unlikely that memorising essays will be of particular help to you in the exam. A better use of your time probably would be to answer essay questions from past exams. If you run out of past exam papers you can always work with a group of other students to prepare and swap essay questions that you have made up yourselves. You can use the topic learning outcomes to develop your essay questions.

Practising essays can help students to revise and think about the information in new ways. However, you don't have to write out essays in full in your essay practice sessions. You may want to do that in the last day or so before the exam, but prior to that, instead of trying to write a full essay when you answer past exam questions, you may find it more useful to practise planning your answer. By this I mean the time that you use to jot down your notes about the structure you will use (e.g. headings), and the bullet points you wish to make in each section. Having done a quick outline of your answer, you are then in a position to go back to your subject notes and see if you have missed out anything that ideally you would need to include. Remember to be critical about any information that you have provided which may be correct but isn't relevant to the question. Take out that information and try again.

Also remember that in your planning during the exam you need to:

- identify what the question is asking you to do (compare and contrast, evaluate, defend a position)
- select what from your studies is relevant to your answer
- determine the structure that you will use in your answer, and
- ascertain what evidence, examples and diagrams are relevant.

The great thing about exam essays is that you don't have to remember exact reference details and you probably aren't expected to provide as much evidence and background detail as you might in an essay not written under exam conditions. Your exam answers will need to be legible though. If you are handwriting exam answers, and you don't write very much any more, it may be helpful to handwrite your practice exams and do so in the time you would have when doing the exam.

Short-answer questions

Short-answer questions really do require a short answer. It is unusual for a short-answer question to be allocated even 15 minutes, unless there are a series of questions within the one question. There are many different types of short-answer question. Some short-answer questions will test your memory while others will determine if you can compare and contrast, evaluate, interpret graphical data and so on. Some questions will ask you to label diagrams correctly (title and legend) and use correct units or symbols in calculations. In every type of short-answer question it's important to interpret the question correctly. A careful reading of each question is essential. You aren't expected to produce long answers that require a structure like an essay. Some examiners will be happy for you to write your short answers as bullet points. Others may prefer you to write sentences. If you know your exam will have short-answer questions in it, you might find it useful to ask your teacher if they will allow bullet-point style answers. If you are asked to do calculations please make sure that you show your working out. The marking scheme that the examiner is using may allow only some of the marks for the right answer, with the rest of the marks being allocated for the work you do to get to the right answer. So you may miss out on some marks even if your final answer is correct. Also, if your answer is wrong, you may still be awarded part marks for showing your correct thinking in earlier steps in your calculation.

Practical exams

Practical exams test your practical skills. There are many, many ways that your practical skills can be tested and many types of learning outcomes that can be tested. For example, the examiner may be testing to see if you can:

- identify parts of equipment, animals, plants
- interpret and manipulate data, e.g. graphical or photographic data
- utilise equipment and take accurate readings
- construct equipment
- make drawings
- carry out a simple experiment or part of an experiment, or
- carry out a procedure successfully.

The learning outcomes related to your practical work will help to guide you in your preparation for a practical exam. My suggestions above for how to proceed in a non-practical exam apply to practical exams. Pacing, answering the question, showing your calculations, etc. are all necessary in the successful completion of a practical exam.

Multiple-choice question (MCQ) exams

MCQ exams generally seek to determine your knowledge and understanding of facts, techniques and concepts and the finer details of your topic of study. They typically comprise a stem that includes the question and a set of answers, some of which aren't correct. The answers that aren't correct are called 'distracters'. There are several keys to taking MCQ exams successfully and I will examine each in turn. Some of these keys are based on the questions and distracters not being well prepared. While we shouldn't rely on this happening, if it does we may be able to use it to our advantage.

1   Preparation – ask if you can see past MCQ exam papers. Working through several papers as part of your preparation will help you to identify the level of detail you need to memorise or understand and it will also help you to become familiar with the type of questions asked. You don't have to have completed all of your revision/study before working through a past paper. Finding out what you don't know can help to guide your study/revision. Try to do the paper under exam conditions and calculate how long you have to do each question, determine which questions to answer first and which to leave until the end. Doing this will help to improve your timing in the exam.

2   For many MCQs it is possible to work out your own answer before looking at the alternatives. Sometimes doing this will help you to choose the correct answer. If calculations are involved, always double-check your calculations even if your answer fits with one of the answers. Teachers will choose distracters that you would calculate if making a small error. Check for any errors.

3   If the question is convoluted, look for the actual question within. For example:

Edinburgh is the capital of Scotland and is found to the east of Glasgow and to the south of Dundee. Scotland borders England. On the East coast of Scotland is the North Sea. To the north of Scotland is the Atlantic and the North Channel is found on the west coast of Scotland. The location of Edinburgh in relation to London is:

a)   north
b)   south
c)   east
d)   west.

The details in the question really aren't giving you any information that is relevant to answering the question. To answer this question you would need to recall a map of the United Kingdom. The question could be reworded to read: Where is Edinburgh located in relation to London? The answer is a).

4   Cross off those distracters that are clearly implausible.

In any given cohort of age-matched teenagers ...

a)   only those who have been directly taught metacognitive skills will possess them
b)   the level of metacognitive skill proficiency will be equivalent across individuals
c)   there will be variability in the extent to which metacognitive skills are possessed
d)   people with a cognitive disability will not be able to learn metacognitive skills.

It only takes one exception for alternatives a), b) and d) to be incorrect. Without knowing anything about the topic, I can determine that c) is more likely to be the correct answer than a), b) or d).

5   Sometimes the correct answer is the longest or most technical.

The term 'side effect' of a drug refers to ...

a)   additional benefits from the drug
b)   the chain effect of drug action
c)   the influence of drugs on crime
d)   any action of a drug in the body other than the one that the doctor wanted the drug to have.

Alternative d) is longer than the rest and very specific and is most likely to be correct.

6   Look for distracters in which the grammar does not match the stem.

Penicillin is obtained from a ...

a)   bacteria
b)   mould
c)   coal-tars
d)   tropical trees.

b) is the only option which is grammatically correct.

7   Look for distracters in which the syntax is different.

The efficacy of a drug ...

a)   determines the potency of the drug if it is a competitive antagonist
b)   at a particular receptor site will always be greater for an agonist than for an antagonist
c)   can be equated with the negative logarithm of the concentration of a drug producing half the maximum response
d)   can be determined from a Scratchard plot
e)   can be measured using the technique of autoradiography.

Alternative b) is of a different syntactic form from the other alternatives and if you don't know the answer, may be more likely to be correct.

8   Look for distracters in which there is a semantic association.

Which of the following diseases is caused by a virus?

a)   gallstones
b)   scarlet fever
c)   typhus fever
d)   typhoid fever
e)   viral pneumonia.

Alternative e) includes the word virus which is found in the question and is therefore most likely to be correct.

9   Look for distracters that are different from the rest.

A drug that blocks the uptake process in sympathetic nerve terminals would be expected to ...

a)   enhance responses to sympathetic nerve stimulation, noradrenaline and tyramine
b)   enhance responses to sympathetic nerve stimulation and noradrenaline but block responses to tyramine
c)   inhibit responses to sympathetic nerve stimulation, noradrenaline and tyramine
d)   enhance responses to guanethidine
e)   enhance responses to isoprenaline.

Alternatives d) and e) stand out as being quite different from a), b) and c) and if there is only one right answer, are likely to be wrong.

10   First impressions aren't always best, i.e. check your paper and if you need to, change your answer, but don't change an answer for the sake of changing it.

11   When in doubt, remember that some examiners tend to use alternatives b) and c) more often than the other alternatives, i.e. if there are four answers you have a twenty-five per cent chance of being right if you guess so don't leave an answer blank.

12   Having calculated how many questions you have to do in every quarter of an hour or so (as demonstrated earlier in the chapter), make sure that you don't spend too long on any one question. If you are having difficulty answering a multiple-choice question, mark what you do know (e.g. any distracters that you have eliminated or the two answers that you think might be right), have a guess at the answer and mark it as one to come back to if you have time at the end of the exam. You will likely get more marks by trying to answer all of the questions than by spending more time on one question and not finishing the exam. Some MCQ exams are designed so that students lose a mark if they get the answer wrong and in this case, you will be best advised not to guess at those questions to which you don't know the answer. The exam paper should say if marks are deducted for incorrect answers.

Failing an exam

Failing an exam isn't actually the end of your world although you may feel that it is. No one wants to fail an exam and yet many people have done so and have lived to tell the tale. If you do fail, you aren't the first to do so and you won't be the last. Exams aren't life-or-death situations. Often you will have the chance to re-sit the exam. Sometimes you may need to take the subject again in the summer semester. If you do need to re-sit an exam or take the subject again, think carefully about why you failed and make sure you have strategies in place to pass the second time. It may help your reflections if you talk with someone else about the strategies you would like to use next time around.

Tips

1   Preparation for exams is usefully done in a planned way throughout the semester.

2   You can choose how much preparation you do for an exam and your choice can be guided by the value of the exam, time needed for other study commitments such as other exams and assignments, and whether you can pass the subject without passing the exam.

3   Pacing yourself during the exam so that you can attempt to answer all questions is an important strategy.

4   Getting a good night's sleep before the exam is likely to be better for your exam success than cramming into the wee hours of the morning.

5   Review tutorials really can be worth attending. It's not necessarily time that you would better spend in revising yourself. The review tutorial may provide you with further insight into what topics to focus on, you may be given information about the make-up of the exam itself, or the teacher may work through specific past exam questions. Making time to attend review tutorials is time well spent.

The next chapter

Increasingly universities provide prospective students with a great deal of choice about where and when they study. Many courses, especially certificates and diplomas, are developed so students can learn entirely online or at a distance. Some courses are blended, providing both online and more traditional face-to-face sessions, perhaps including intensive weekends or weeks of study. Studying online is both similar to and different from studying on campus. In the next chapter those differences and similarities are explored. The chapter provides the reader with a clear idea of the responsibilities of an online student and the strategies that can be used to study successfully.

7   Learning online

Peter Ling

Learning outcomes

By the end of this chapter readers are expected to be able to:

*   identify what they are expected to do as students in a subject that is offered wholly or partly online
*   devise strategies for learning effectively online, and
*   identify resources that will help them with learning online.

Introduction

As a student in an accredited health care course you are more and more likely to find that some component of your study is offered online. The reasons for this range from providing place and time flexibility for students with multiple commitments, through using the technology for information sharing and communications which is preferred by an ever increasing segment of the population, to dealing with human and physical resource issues within teaching institutions. While we all use electronic communications in some form or another, many of us have not used it to learn in an accredited course. That can raise some questions. How can learning online substitute for a classroom? What are students expected to do when a subject is offered online? Are there successful strategies for learning online? Is there anybody or anything out there to support the student?

In this chapter we will address these questions and prepare you to learn effectively online and to make the most of the choices and resources it offers.

What is learning online?

The basic learning activities conducted in classrooms can be provided for online: lectures, tutorials, seminars, informal discussion, chat, guidance to reference material. You miss some of the face-to-face cues that help with interpersonal interaction and you may not have access to some of the physical materials and tools that we are used to using, for instance in laboratory settings. On the other hand you are not limited by what is in the teaching space – the people or the material things. You have access to online library resources and the internet, which is increasingly the place we turn to for information and interaction. And when it comes to laboratory work you may miss out on the real thing but may have virtual substitutes that you can't break and can test to the limits as you learn – the classic instance is the flight simulator.

When we ask 'what is learning online?' we need to take account of the answer to the question 'what is learning?' In higher education learning involves more than acquiring information that can be regurgitated in exams. It involves coming to grips with sophisticated concepts, developing complex skills and, in the health field, developing propensities to act in desired ways. If the learning outcomes of a subject are well written they will give you an indication of what you should be able to do on completion of the subject. The learning objectives might indicate that on completion of the subject you will be able to analyse some situation, be able to explain some concept, be able to perform some skilled behaviour. To be able to demonstrate that you have met these outcomes requires more than learning some information by heart. It requires a deeper level of understanding. This is likely to be assisted by active involvement in the learning context – by questioning, discussing, analysing, concept mapping, or thinking of instances or examples that resonate with you. The same applies to learning online. Active involvement of this sort with online materials will help you get to the underlying concepts. Using online communications facilities to discuss concepts with others and to raise questions will have you actively involved in your learning and improve chances of success.

Models

There is no unitary answer to what is learning online. There are various approaches, models and mixes, that range from everything online to blended learning.

Everything online includes teaching materials, learning resources, communication with teachers, networking with fellow learners, quizzes, and assessment.

Blended learning may include lectures online, in print or in audio-visual form, tutorial materials online, discussion online, assignments online, group work online. These may be supplemented by face-to-face classes, workshops or informal groups or perhaps by intensive periods of attendance.

Responsibility of students and teachers

Teachers

Teachers are responsible for structuring learning experiences, providing guidance and resources or leading students to resources. They may structure online discussion, monitor it and encourage contribution. Teachers specify assessment expectations and facilitate completion, provide feedback on progress, and may prompt students who are falling behind. The teacher can post announcements online, for example on course administration matters or on the next phase of a study programme.

Is the teacher there to answer your questions? Ultimately yes but questions from students via phone or email can place an unreasonable load on teachers with large numbers of students online so teachers may employ strategies that will provide answers to questions without having to answer each individually, just as they may do in class. They may suggest for instance that students place their questions in an online discussion forum. This provides the opportunity for other students to answer the question or at least for other students to see the response of the teacher, avoiding the need to deal with the same question multiple times.

Students

Students need to determine what is expected of them and how the learning is expected to occur in the particular subject. In some cases the expectations of students will be specified. If not, here are some guidelines. Read directly provided material. Select from other reference material to meet your specific needs. Interact with teachers and with fellow students through the means available, e.g. online discussion. You may also wish to use facilities available to network informally with other students through email, discussion and chat. Revisit the online subject site regularly so that you are aware of new announcements from the teacher and new contributions to online discussions lodged by the teacher and other students.

Getting started

If you are new to learning online you may want answers to some basic questions.

- How do I find the subject website?
- How do I log on?
- What do I do next?

You may find that the teachers involved and technicians responsible for online provision are so used to online teaching and learning that they are more concerned with enhancing teaching materials or refining technical capabilities than focusing on basic access needs. Nevertheless you can be sure that some of the basics will have been addressed because these questions do not have intuitive answers – everyone needs some guidance here.

How do I find the website for the subject?

Online tuition generally involves the use of a learning online management system such as WebCT or Blackboard. The subject website might look something like the one in Figure 7.1. These sites provide a structure for the study of the subject. In Figure 7.1 you can see eleven boxes or tabs on the left-hand side (announcements, unit outline, etc.). Each of these tabs leads to an area of the site in which a student can locate online teaching materials, links to reference material, the online discussion board, information about assessment requirements and possibly assessment tasks online and results or grades. It is not necessarily a one-stop shop but it will be the hub for your learning online experience. As such you can expect that its URL will be included in any printed course material or on the website for the institution or teaching department. If you cannot find it you will have to call and ask if there is a website and if so ask for the address or the URL. The address might look something like http://www.universityname.ac.uk/.

When I get there how do I log on?

Online learning websites generally have restricted access. Obtaining access will usually involve a username and password. These will need to be supplied by your higher education institution. If you don't have them the institution may have an information technologies unit with an online service desk that may be able to help you. Otherwise ring the department offering your course of study. Detailed log-on instructions are generally provided on the web page where you log on.

Strategies for learning online

One thing for the traditional lecture and tutorial approach – it gets timetabled into your week and you organise at least part of your life around it. Sometimes you notice the difference between the regularly scheduled components such as the lectures, and the reading and assignments you are

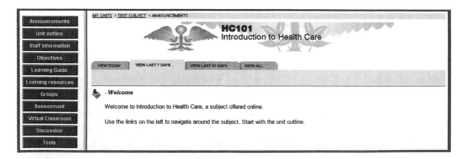

Figure 7.1 An example of a home page of a subject website

supposed to do in your own time. It takes another level of organisation and self-discipline to deal with the aspects of study that you need to do in your own time. When it comes to learning online it is often as though all of this study is in the second category where you need to determine where you are going to fit it into your life. Leaving assignments to the last minute is generally not a good strategy (Chapter 5) and neither is putting off online involvement in the course. In fact the longer you leave it the harder it is to get started. Get in as early as you can. Ring up or email if you think you should have access to a subject and cannot open it online. There are several things that can go wrong with access from the whole class level to the individual, including enrolment issues, technical issues and the teacher forgetting to turn the site on.

Get an overview of what is on the site

Learn the navigation. Look for directions from the teacher about what is provided and how you are expected to use it. Find the assessment requirements and when they are due. Work back from that to create a schedule for yourself on which aspects of the subject you need to have covered and what learning activities you need to have engaged with in order to meet the due dates.

How to use tuition material

The website is likely to provide some text material in the form of web pages. It may provide online lectures in audio or video format, lecture notes, and PowerPoint slides. These provide the basic materials that substitute for what you could expect to receive in a class. It is not just a matter of reading these materials; it is a matter of being able to identify the main points that will contribute to your learning. You may want to make your own set of notes on the topic informed by these materials.

How to use other resources

A higher education course usually involves accessing resources beyond lecture notes and the material provided online. This does not mean reading everything that is referred to in its entirety. Be selective. Use the tables of contents in books and reports, book indexes, and online search facilities. If you are searching for information online use the Google 'advanced search' where you can be more specific about what you are looking for.

How to use communications facilities

Online you can use email for direct one-to-one communication but generally, where an online learning management system is used, you are expected to use the discussion facility on the system so that all students can take note of issues and make responses. Some learning management systems allow students and teachers to email others enrolled in the subject. When they do this the mail goes to your student email address rather than to your usual email address. It can be a good idea to redirect your student email to your preferred email address to save monitoring two locations. You can do this by setting up a 'rule' in your student email account to the effect that all mail received at this address will be forwarded to your preferred address. Your university's information technology services will be able to advise you how to do this.

Online learning may make use of discussion, which generally refers to asynchronous interaction – that is, participants do not need to be online at the same time. Online discussion may be required or optional. It may be part of group work. Remember that it takes someone to make the first move. If that has not been structured into the online activity take the initiative – it gives you first go at determining the focus of the discussion. Other forms of asynchronous communication used are wikis – sites for groups to interact in building up materials – and blogs – websites for journaling and other forms of personal expression open to the public or to a select group. You should be instructed on how to access any of these facilities that are available for your subject.

Communication may also involve chat and other forms of synchronous media where the interaction between participants occurs at a specific time or in 'real time' as some would say. This can include telephone conferencing or web conferencing. Web conferencing can include exchange using text (chat), voice, or video cameras. It can include shared 'white board' space, which allows participants to share in drafting drawings as well as text. Synchronous exchanges may be used while an online lecture is running. Another form of synchronous exchange is the use of virtual spaces, such as Second Life where learning resources may be available and students and teachers may communicate using avatars or a representation of themselves. Again you should be instructed on how to access any of these facilities that are available for your subject.

Group work online

Working in groups is a normal part of face-to-face tuition. Sometimes it occurs informally but it is often a formal part of a subject and involves assessment tasks. You will need to participate in formal groups where this is part of the course but you can also find ways to communicate informally with groups. Sometimes specific roles are assigned to members of the groups and this will indicate who is responsible for getting it started but if this is not the case there are advantages in taking the initiative and getting the group active. Early participation can give you a voice in defining the group's operation and roles.

Working in groups involves the use of synchronous and asynchronous communications discussed above under strategies for learning online. It may also involve use of a wiki or a file exchange provided by an online learning management system. File exchange allows a document to be lodged online and accessed and modified by members of the group to produce a group outcome.

Blended learning

Blended learning refers to the use of online and other electronic media in conjunction with face-to-face tuition. It may involve a crafted package of learning activities where each component – face-to-face and online – is required or it may provide options where students can choose the ways in which they want to learn.

Use of multiple types of media

Blended learning may make use of a range of media. Audio and audio-visual material, such as video recorded lectures, may be made available synchronously in remote locations or may be made available asynchronously on CD or DVD or online. Online this material may take the form of:

- files that you can download to your computer (but note that this can soon use up your disk space and you may need to delete the files regularly)
- streaming media that plays on your computer but is not downloaded. This may or may not allow you to pause, which is a desirable feature of online learning media
- podcasts that can provide you with the latest in a series of lectures if you subscribe to them. You can podcast to a computer or to a video ipod or the like. A video ipod gives a small image but gives more time and place flexibility.

Online or CD and DVD learning materials may include what is often referred to as multimedia, that is, electronic material including text, video, audio, animations. It may include electronic simulations and games.

Blended learning may involve asynchronous discussion, wikis and blogs. It may also make use of various synchronous forms of communication referred to above under strategies for learning online. Media may include online quizzes, tasks and other activities.

Your task as a student is to become acquainted with what is on offer and to use it to support your learning. If your subject is one in which multiple types of media are available then, unless you are told you must use them all, select the forms that best suit you. Use multiple forms if you are having difficulty with a concept or skill.

Purpose-specific modes of study

Blended learning is often structured to use select media for specific purposes. For instance the key information on topics, which was typically presented in lectures, may be placed online instead. Wider reading and other learning resources may also be online. Face-to-face classes may be used to pursue tutorial questions and provide for interaction between teachers and students and/or for laboratory work. The expectation of students may be spelt out; you may be told that you are expected to attend classes and complete certain parts of your study online. If it is not spelt out then work out for yourself whether what is on offer is designed to provide you with learning options or is designed as a complete suite where you need all components to ensure success.

Learning options

Blended learning may be designed to provide learning options for those with time and place constraints, including those who prefer to vary their pace of study and work in intensive bursts. It may be designed to cater for students with particular learning needs. For students with disabilities learning online may be a good option. For students from non-English-speaking backgrounds learning online reduces the chances of mishearing, it provides accurate notes, and provides the opportunity to revise material.

It is not a case of 'either/or'. Where learning options are provided you can attend classes and use online materials. For all students, including those who attend class, online materials provide the chance to revise, which is a popular use of online resources.

In making a decision about attending sessions that are also available online in video, audio or print form think about some of the advantages that can arise from attendance. These include: motivation from live presentations by the teacher; the chance to interact with the teacher and discuss issues with other students; seeing visual materials that may not be replicated online; and being able to ask questions about assessment and administrative matters as well as about the subject matter. Attendance provides the discipline of setting aside time for study. On the other hand don't let attendance substitute for learning. The deep learning expected in higher education requires that you internalise the subject. It requires more than having heard someone speak about it in class.

Related to this, for some students listening and taking thoughtful notes as a lecturer speaks can really assist them to grasp the key points; for many students note taking and learning are mutually exclusive activities. If you fall into the second category look to the online resources provided. Teachers often provide lecture notes and/or PowerPoint slides online. If they do you can focus your attention on the key concepts in class rather than on note taking. If slides or notes are available online prior to the class print them out and jot down points during the lecture that help to explain the concepts to you. If teachers make a habit of posting material online after the event you may be able to persuade them that it would be of more value to you to have the material in advance.

Getting help and support

There is often a range of types of help for students available. We have dealt with academic support specific to your subject above. Associated with this is help with study skills, such as how to write essays or how to cite references. This is often pertinent to people returning to study. The university may have study skills advisers but there is also help available through a number of websites online, e.g. Startup 2008 at Curtin University: http://startup.curtin.edu.au/study/. Related support available may include counselling for personal issues relating to study.

University libraries, which used to be envisaged as buildings housing books and journals, are increasingly the online gateway to learning resources. Libraries generally provide clear instructions to accessing resources online. In some cases you may need a username and password for access. Contact the library helpdesk or a reference librarian if you need assistance.

Universities generally provide assistance with technical advice relating to learning online, including equipment requirements and setting up equipment, through information technology units, which are likely to have a telephone or online helpdesk or at least email support. For help with software such as online learning management systems look for a help tab or button. In some cases they may simply be identified by '?'.

Conclusion

Looking back at the learning outcomes for this chapter, seek out the expectations of you as a student in your particular subject. They should be defined on the website for the subject. Ask the questions you need answered if they are not. Where a subject is offered in blended form, ascertain whether you are expected to attend classes and to deal with everything online or whether there are options. If there are options choose what suits your learning needs. You may still wish to do the lot. Devise your own strategies for working online but remember that it requires greater self-discipline than attending regular classes. Get going early in the piece, set up a study schedule that will get you there before the end of the study period. Remember that there is a world of resources online that can help you with your study of the subject; some are provided within universities such as library resources and study advisory services, and some are reached through the wider realms of the internet that may be accessed through search engines and Wikipedia.

The next chapter

The topic of the next chapter is group work and the book ends with this chapter for several reasons, one of which is the importance of group work to health care professionals in their everyday work. The usefulness of the ideas and strategies discussed in the group work chapter will extend beyond your student days and well into your career as a health care professional.

8   Working in groups

Jane Fowler, Amanda Gudmundsson and Leanne Whicker

Learning outcomes

By the end of this chapter readers are expected to be able to:

- work effectively and productively in a group
- set goals, share expectations and develop a contract for working in a group
- make efficient use of planning and meeting time to achieve goals
- understand the value of balancing task and maintenance group behaviours, and
- recognise and develop the contributions that they make to a group.

Introduction

This chapter is a condensation of a guide written by the chapter authors for both university teachers and students (Fowler *et al.*, 2006). All page references given in this chapter are to this guide, unless otherwise stated.

University students often work in groups. It may be a formal group (i.e. one that has been formed for a group presentation, writing a report, or completing a project) or an informal group (i.e. some students have decided to form a study group or undertake research together). Whether formal or informal, this chapter aims to make working in groups easier for you.

Health care professionals also often work in groups. Yes, working in groups will extend well beyond your time at university. In fact, the skills and abilities to work effectively in groups are some of the most sought-after attributes in health care professionals. It seems obvious, then, that taking the opportunity to develop and enhance your skills and abilities for working in groups is a wise choice.

> At work, most major decisions are made by groups ... [This is because groups can achieve many tasks that an individual cannot complete by

working alone]. Groups of people with complementary skills can work more effectively on large and complex tasks. 'Synergy' is the term used to describe the ability of a group to achieve more than the sum of its parts (i.e. more than the total of the group members' individual abilities). However, groups have to be understood and managed if they are to be effective. Just bringing people together does not guarantee they will be successful.

(pp. 7–8)

What's in it for me?

We know that students often don't like working in groups. This is usually because of negative group experiences caused by inadequate forming and contracting, insufficient planning and organising, and inability to overcome difficulties that arise along the way. Some preparatory work can help you prevent and overcome these negative experiences.

This will take some time and effort on your part. How much time and effort will depend on each individual and group. However, be assured that proactive time and effort invested in the early stages of group formation usually result in a reduction of reactive time and effort needed to overcome problems and difficulties that might occur later in the group's life together. It is important to remember that each group experience, whether it seems positive or negative at the time, can be reflected on and learnt from to enhance future group experiences.

You can also learn a lot about yourself from working in groups – your strengths, preferences, personality characteristics and values, and how they influence and are influenced by other people. Working in groups provides ongoing opportunities for self-reflection and learning. Being part of an effective group can be stimulating, enjoyable and rewarding for all group members.

Effective groups

Effective and productive groups can be created, developed and maintained. However, it doesn't just happen; it takes time, effort and commitment. Most individuals want to be 'good' group members and can enjoy the experience of group work.

In our experience of working with various groups over many years, we have found that some of the characteristics of effective groups are:

- shared aims and objectives
- clear direction and purpose
- active and genuine participation by all members in group activities
- shared expectations about contribution and effort
- commitment to the group

- shared responsibility for group process and outcomes
- effective decision-making processes
- open communication and sharing of information
- expression of feelings and disagreements
- an honest and open approach to dealing with concerns and issues
- a climate that does not stifle individuality, and
- a balanced approach to satisfying individual and group needs.
  (Adapted from Fowler *et al.*, 2006; Mullins, 2002; Wood *et al.*, 2004)

Task and maintenance

Generally speaking, an effective group is one that achieves its goals (i.e. gets the tasks done) while taking care of the relationships among its members in the process. Another way of saying this is, that effective groups know to look beyond 'what' they are doing (the task they are completing) to 'how' they are doing it (the process in which they are engaging).

In order to be able to 'get the task done' while taking care of group members in the process, groups need to engage in what Tyson (1998) referred to as 'task' and 'maintenance' behaviours.

Task behaviours are necessary for ensuring that the group is able to perform well, be productive, achieve its goals and get the job done.

Maintenance behaviours focus on how the group members go about working on their task, i.e. caring for each other, showing concern for feelings, providing opportunities for each group member to contribute and maintaining healthy relationships in the group.

We know that when you have a group project to complete, you really just want to 'get on with it'. In most groups, members tend to emphasise the importance of this task dimension over the maintenance dimension. Tyson (1998) pointed out that emphasis of one over the other is likely to lead to frustration, discontent or withdrawal. Effective groups, however, strike an appropriate balance between focusing on the task and maintaining relationships and concern for group members. Striking this balance is likely to lead to a more cohesive group which in turn will enhance performance. We will talk a little bit more about task and maintenance behaviours later in this chapter.

Forming a group

If you have the opportunity to choose your group,

> it might be wise to give consideration to a range of issues that can impact on the functioning of a group. Rather than provide a list of what you should or should not do, we raise questions for you to consider. You may find that some or none of them are important to you, or you might have other issues that are equally as important. You may

find it helpful to first reflect on these questions for yourself, and then discuss with others.

- *Diversity* – is it desirable or important that you have a gender, age, or ethnic mix in your group? Why?
- *Timetable* – how does your 'life timetable' fit in with the other potential members of your group? That is, realistically, how easy will it be for you to meet or make contact? And is this acceptable to all members?
- *Location* – is where you live or work likely to impact on time and place for group meetings?
- *Topic* – is forming a group around a particular topic/task more important than forming around issues such as diversity, commitment, location, timetable? Why?
- *Grade level desired* – if a group mark is to be awarded, how will students [shooting] for a higher grade impact on students who are happy with a pass grade and vice-versa? Why?
- *Friendship* – is working with friends desirable or important or challenging? Why?
- Are there any other issues that are important for you, or potential members of your group, in determining group formation?

Whether you had the opportunity to self-select into your group or whether you were appointed to your group, early planning work is the most effective way to help you avoid potential pitfalls.

(p. 11)

Each of you will have some assumptions about what to expect from the group, and what you expect to give or contribute to the group. 'We recommend that you spend some time exploring these assumptions and expectations, and get to know each other. This is important for your group's development regardless of whether some or all of you have worked together before' (p. 12).

Getting to know your group members

Each time a group forms they are a new group, regardless of whether none, some, or all have worked together previously. Group members learn from their experiences and develop new knowledge, skills, and abilities that need to be considered in the forming and developing process. In some cases, negative experiences may not have been dealt with effectively and 'baggage' may be transferred to the new group. In most cases, the reason for forming the group will have changed (probably a new task) which will require appropriate contracting and negotiation. Therefore, it is important that the new group's identity is recognised with appropriate forming, contracting, and relationship building processes.

In the early stages of development, group members are attempting to become better acquainted with each other in addition to becoming orientated with the task about to be undertaken. In order to facilitate the team building process groups can engage in activities and processes that encourage communication and interaction which will help members to become more comfortable with one another and begin feeling like they are part of a team.

(p. 17)

One way of doing this is to think about the ways you prefer to function as a group member. Jot down a few notes for each of the prompts below. Then, share your responses with the other members of your group.

- What I would like to get out of this group
- How I will ensure everyone gets the opportunity to participate
- How I would address problems in the group
- How I will go about giving positive/negative feedback to others in the group
- My most positive and most negative group experience
- What I would like to get out of this course
- One of the skills I would really like to learn is …
- At the end of this group experience I would like to be able to …
- Other things I wish to discuss …

(p. 14)

Clarifying expectations and setting ground rules

You will have implicit (or unstated) understandings and expectations about what you and others 'give to' and 'receive from' the group. So will your other group members.

For example, we all have expectations about how much work we will be required to do, the amount of emotional energy we need to invest, and how we will be included in the group's activities. If one or more members fail to comply with the unstated expectations of others it could impact on the relationships in the group – and the group's effectiveness. However, making explicit (or stating) your understandings and expectations will help to clarify and develop a shared understanding of how the group will work together.

(p. 20)

- What are the expectations that we have of each other?
- Do I have other priorities that may impact on my contribution to the group (e.g., university/work/family/sporting/community commitments)?

- What academic results do I wish to achieve and what level of time and effort am I willing to devote to achieving that outcome?
- Do I expect this group to be social and friendly or more formal and business like?
- Are there some other expectations we should talk about?

(p. 19)

Before your group begins working on the content of your project it is important that the group discusses and negotiates the ground rules, or the process, that the group will follow when working together. In order to reach your group's goal/s, it is important to establish standards and expectations regarding individual contribution and performance. With these expectations in mind you can begin to discuss and negotiate the ground rules that are necessary to help guide and facilitate the effective functioning of your group. The following questions are designed to help prompt your thinking and generate a list of ground rules. Discuss and negotiate the rules proposed to ensure that all members of the group are satisfied and committed to them. These ground rules will guide your interactions while in this group.

- How are we going to organise group meetings – what procedures need to be put in place?
- How are we going to share the workload?
- How are we going to monitor whether we are achieving our group's goal/s?
- If I/we become dissatisfied with how we are going as a group, what are some possible ways to solve the problem?
- What expectations do we want to set regarding attendance at group meetings?
- What are we going to do about a group member who doesn't contribute their fair share of the work?

The ground rules you ... set may need changing and adjusting as the group progresses and matures. So, [from time-to-time], review your ground rules and consider whether the group is adhering to them. If members leave your group, or new members join, it will be necessary to revisit these ground rules. Changes to the group membership are significant in the development of the group, so we suggest that the group should re-form and re-contract when a member leaves or joins.

(p. 21)

Group contact list

You may decide that every member of the group should be able to contact every other member. In this case, share with the group members your preferred contact details. If you are aware of any constraints or

Table 8.1 Group contact list

Group member	Phone	E-mail	Preferences/ constraints
1			
2			
3			
4			
5			
6			

restrictions regarding your details, [it would be useful to] inform the others. For instance, perhaps you work every Monday evening, or are only able to access your e-mail on particular days, or prefer that people didn't call you before or after a certain time of the day. Perhaps you may already know that you will be away for a certain period of time during the group's task.

Being clear and open [from the start] about your contact arrangements will help prevent misunderstanding and frustration in the future when group members are trying to contact you.

(p. 22)

Goal setting and planning

Your group is likely to have been established so that you may work on a task or specific project together, so you will need to identify what you wish to achieve by setting goals for the group and plan how your group is going to achieve its goals. The extent of your goal setting and project planning will depend upon the size of the project. You will need to make some choices about how much planning is needed. For example, you may be required to work as a group for the duration of the semester (on one or a number of tasks). Alternatively, you may be working on a group presentation for a class in three weeks' time. So, depending on the complexity of your task/project, and your group's needs, you will decide how much planning is necessary. Here we describe a process that can assist with your planning.

Discuss the following questions:

- What is the task that our group has to complete?
- What is expected of us?
- How much work will this involve?
- What questions do we have about the task?

Table 8.2 Goal setting

Tasks/activities (plus resources)	Task priority and sequence	Estimated time for completing task	Group members(s) responsible

... Identify the list of specific tasks and activities that need to be accomplished. Try and be as specific as possible. This may take some time, particularly if it is the first time you have worked on this type of project.

As you identify your list of tasks and activities, consider whether there are any specific resources that will be needed in order to complete them (e.g., library facilities, internet access, etc.).

You may need to revisit this list as you progress through the project and identify additional work that needs to be undertaken ... Determine the priorities and sequence of activities. Consider whether some activities need to be finished before you can commence others or whether some activities can be done at the same time ... Schedule the estimated amount of time necessary to complete each task or activity.

(pp. 27–28)

Decide who is responsible for the various tasks or activities, so the workload can be distributed equally. Finally, co-ordinate the various tasks and activities that members are completing in order to meet the project or assignment deadline.

A simple table is provided above to help you with your planning process. Remember that even the most well thought-out plan can lack some details, so planning may continue throughout the project.

Organising group meetings

Your group meetings will tend to be more effective if they have some form of structure and organisation rather than being informal chats. Your group will need to identify the level of structure most appropriate for your purpose.

You may wish to assign roles such as 'leader', 'note-taker' and 'time-keeper' – and rotate these roles at each meeting.

> The person *leading* the meeting assists the group to achieve its meeting objectives by ensuring that all agenda items [or important points] are covered, [elicits] contributions from all members, helps to keep the discussions focused on the topic but at the same time is careful not to inhibit creative processes, and summarises the ideas and decisions the group makes. The *note-taker* keeps a record of the group's discussions and the decisions being made throughout the meeting ... The *time-keeper* is responsible for monitoring the time taken to discuss agenda items [so that everything gets covered]...
>
> [You will need to] decide on the length of time for each meeting and the frequency of meetings to be scheduled for the duration of the project or assignment. Be aware that at the start of the project your group may need to meet more frequently and for longer periods of time in comparison to the meetings necessary towards the conclusion of the project ...
>
> Plan ahead for the next meeting. What does your group need to discuss? What information do you need to bring to the meeting? It is important to use meeting time efficiently, so be prepared and think about the outcomes your group wants to achieve from each meeting ...
>
> After your group has met it is useful to evaluate the effectiveness of your meeting process. Changes to the meeting process (i.e. the structure and organisation) [may be needed] to ensure that future meetings are more effective ... [Ask yourselves questions such as]:
>
> * Before the meeting began were all members clear about what the meeting was meant to achieve?
> * Did we achieve our overall meeting objective?
> * Did we discuss [everything that needed to be discussed]?
> * Were our discussions focused and a good use of time?
> * Did we identify the tasks that need to be completed before our next meeting and who is responsible for completing these tasks?
> * Have we identified [what needs to be discussed at our next meeting, and where and when it will be]?
> * Was our meeting both productive and enjoyable?
>
> (pp. 31–32; italics added)

Working together as a group

The task of any group is usually easy to identify. The group members may meet regularly to discuss their project, assign tasks to individuals or sub-groups, and monitor their progress towards achieving the end result. If you were observing these groups in action, you could see the outcomes of this type of activity. However, there is another type of activity that is rarely explicitly observed or discussed, mainly because the group members are focused on the task itself. This activity is the group process, [i.e.] *how* the group goes about working on their task.

Tyson (1998, p. 65) described group process as 'how the group is behaving from moment to moment, the sequence of activities, interactions and movements of the members as they go about their work and relate to each other'. Tyson also said that group 'process is [the] dynamic, continuous and ever-changing' levels of energy, mood, noise, vitality and pace as the group members interact with each other. The group process has a critical influence on the success of the group.

(p. 35)

Group members can identify and describe these changes in the group process by observing what is going on in the group. In other words, what task and maintenance behaviours are being performed (remember we introduced these concepts earlier in the chapter) – and by whom? Observing what is happening in the group is a way of bringing into awareness aspects about the group's process that can be very helpful if, say, the group gets 'stuck', or cannot agree on a decision. Below is a short (but certainly not exhaustive) list of group behaviours that may be observed.

Task behaviours [ensure that the group achieves its goals, i.e. gets the job done].

- *Initiating* – start[ing] the discussion; propos[ing] tasks
- *Information or Opinion seeking* – [asking] for ideas, suggestions, opinions, or concerns
- *Information or Opinion giving* – [giving] ideas, suggestions, opinions or concerns
- *Clarifying* – giving examples; [seeking] more information or elaboration to clear up confusion
- *Summarising* – [pulling] together what has been said; [restating] ideas; [organising] related information
- *Implementing* – [putting] into action the ideas [or] decisions of the group
- *Creating/Innovating* – [generating] or [bringing] in new ideas, concepts or ways of thinking about the task

Maintenance behaviours ensure that the group maintains healthy and/or harmonious relationships while getting the job done.

- *Encouraging* – ... responsive to ideas; reinforces suggestions; uses body language to encourage others
- *Approval* – accepts or approves of others' participation
- *Sharing feelings* – expresses group feelings, or moods; is aware of shifts in energy or tone; encourages others to share feelings

- *Harmonising/Compromising* – seeks to reduce tension; works out disagreements; looks for compromise
- *Gatekeeping* – helps others to participate, encourages non-contributors; controls dominating speakers

(Adapted from Scholtes, 1992, cited in Fowler *et al.*, 2006, p. 38; italics added)

Asking yourselves (either individually or as a group) whether these and other necessary behaviours are being performed – and by whom – can be a very useful way of helping your group move forward. It is relatively simple. For example, next time you are in a group, observe which group member/s talk the most, talk the least, offer ideas and suggestions, encourage or discourage, participate, and whose opinion seems to have the most influence. An observation that not all members of the group are participating during an idea generation or brainstorming session can be brought to the attention of the group. This observation can then be the basis for discussion (there may be a number of reasons for lack of contribution) and action (what, if anything, do we need to do differently?).

Facilitating the group

Some groups may have a formal leader or facilitator (either assigned or elected) to co-ordinate, unite and direct the efforts of the group. Other groups may be self-directing and collaborative and prefer to share the facilitation and leadership. Most groups at university will not formalise the role of the leader and will need all members to display leadership and facilitation behaviours at one time or another.

Some people are uncomfortable taking on this role because of a lack of confidence or experience, or because they associate the word 'leader' with being 'bossy' or dominant. We need to get something straight – leadership is not a dirty word. It is how someone goes about the role of leader that determines whether they are 'bossy' or not. Another way of saying this is that a leader can choose to be 'bossy' or 'facilitative'. Also, one single member does not have to undertake this role at every meeting. It may be that the group chooses to nominate the facilitator at the start of each meeting and rotate the role throughout the life of the group.

So, it might be helpful to think of this role as 'facilitator' rather than 'leader'. The purpose of the facilitator role is to ensure the group is moving toward its goals (the task) while paying adequate attention to how it functions (maintenance). The facilitator elicits ideas and encourages group discussion. You don't have to be an expert – it may be as simple as asking 'Where should we start today?', 'What do you think, Tyron?', or 'Do we need to spend more time on this?' Equally, it could be as simple as contributing comments such as 'OK, it seems we have three key ideas: how should we go about making a decision on this?' or 'Well, it sounds like we've decided to ABC; is everyone ready to move on to XYZ?' Thus, you are simply facilitating the group's process.

Becoming an effective facilitator requires practice and concentration. Although it may be something you are not comfortable with at first, good facilitation skills are useful in any work setting.

Feedback in groups

When working as members of a group it is often necessary to provide feedback to one another. It is through this feedback that individuals and the group can enhance effectiveness by consolidating behaviours that produce success and minimising behaviours that impede the group's progress.

Giving and receiving feedback are important skills to develop for your future professional career. Feedback to and from supervisors, subordinates, co-workers and clients is a regular part of everyday work life. Unfortunately, feedback is often poorly communicated resulting in heightened emotion and anxiety. Poorly communicated feedback frequently creates greater problems than the feedback was intended to solve. Therefore, in order to work effectively in a group setting it is essential that you learn to give and receive feedback sensitively and skilfully.

(p. 41)

The following ideas about how to give and receive feedback are taken from Fowler *et al.*, 2006, pp. 41–44.

How to give feedback

Start with the positive

Most people respond well to encouragement. It can help the receiver to hear first what you liked about what they have done or accomplished before providing negative feedback ...

Be specific

Avoid general or vague comments which are not very useful ... Statements such as 'You were brilliant!' or 'It was awful', may be pleasant or dreadful to hear, but they do not give enough detail to be useful sources of learning. Try to pinpoint what the person did that led you to use the label 'brilliant' or 'awful' ...

Refer to the behaviour that can be changed, rather than the person

It is important to describe what a person does that you like or dislike rather than comment on what you think of them as a person. It is not likely to be helpful to give a person feedback about something over which they have no choice or control ...

Offer alternatives

If you do offer negative feedback, then do not simply criticise, but suggest what the person could have done differently. The feedback then becomes constructive negative feedback through the use of a positive suggestion ...

Be descriptive rather than evaluative

Describe to the person what you saw or heard and the effect it had on you rather than merely providing a 'good' or 'bad' judgement ...

Own the feedback

It can be easy to say to the other person 'You are ...', suggesting that you are offering a universally agreed opinion about that person. However, all we are really entitled to give is our own experience of that person at a particular time. It is also important that we take responsibility for the feedback we offer. Beginning the feedback with 'I' or 'In my opinion' is a way of avoiding the impression of being the giver of 'cosmic judgements' about the other person ...

Leave the recipient with a choice

Feedback that demands change or is imposed heavily on the other person may invite resistance. Skilled feedback offers people information about themselves in a way that leaves them with a choice about whether to act on it or not. It can help to examine the consequences of any decision to change or not to change, but does not involve prescribing change ...

Choose the right time and place to give the feedback

Generally, feedback is more helpful when given as soon as possible after the event. However, exceptions to this guideline would be when you might be so angry that you would be unlikely to give constructive feedback, or when the recipient is too upset, busy or tired to receive the feedback. It is also worthwhile to consider whether you are in the right place to provide feedback, for instance whether the feedback should be provided in a public or private forum?

Follow up on the feedback

When you have given constructive feedback and this has resulted in a positive change in the receiver's behaviour, it is valuable to notice and acknowledge the behaviour change.

Think what it says about you

Feedback is likely to say as much about the giver as the receiver. It will say a good deal about your values, and what you focus on in others. Therefore we can learn about ourselves if we listen to the feedback we give others.

How to receive feedback

Listen to the feedback rather than immediately rejecting or arguing with it

Negative feedback can be uncomfortable to hear, but we may benefit from it. Likewise, we can benefit from receiving feedback about positive aspects of our behaviour. People do have their opinions about you and will have their perceptions of your behaviour, and it can help to be aware of those. However, do remember that you are also entitled to your opinion and you may choose to ignore the feedback as being of little significance, irrelevant, or referring to behaviour which for some other reason you wish to maintain.

Be clear about what is being said

Try to avoid jumping to conclusions or becoming immediately defensive, otherwise people may cut down their feedback or you may not be able to use it fully. Make sure you understand the feedback before you respond to it. A useful technique can be to paraphrase or repeat the feedback, to check that you have understood.

Check it out with others rather than relying on only one source

If we rely on one source, then we may imagine that the individual's opinion is shared by everybody. However, if we check with others, we may find that they experience us differently and we will have a more balanced view of ourselves, which can keep the feedback in proportion.

Ask for the feedback you want but do not get

Feedback is important. Ask for feedback that is not forthcoming. Sometimes we do get feedback but it is restricted to one aspect of our behaviour. We may have to request further feedback we would find useful but do not get.

Decide what you will do as a result of the feedback

Each of us needs to know how other people experience us to extend our self-awareness. We can use feedback to help our own development. When we receive it, we can assess its value, the consequences of ignoring or using it, and finally decide what we will do as a result of it. Try not to over- or under-react to feedback. However, if we do not make decisions on the basis of the feedback, then it can be wasted.

Thank the person giving the feedback

Finally, thank the person for giving the feedback. Providing feedback can be difficult and may not have been easy for the person to give. It is a valuable practice to reinforce in any relationship.

Generating ideas and making decisions

At various times throughout your group's project, you may need to generate ideas. These ideas may be in relation to the task you are completing (e.g., the topic on which you will work, how you will arrange a group presentation, or how you might approach an assignment) or in relation to how your group works (e.g., how you will divide the tasks, or where and how frequently you will meet). It is important that all members have an opportunity to share their ideas. All ideas should be considered and explored before making decisions about how to proceed ...

There are numerous methods of generating ideas, each with implications for the group ... For example, if you need to generate ideas on a single concept problem, such as choosing a title for your group presentation, you might adopt *the brainstorming* method to generate as many ideas as possible. However, if it is a more complex issue, such as an overall design for a workshop you are going to conduct, then you might adopt *the nominal group technique* [i.e. members work on the problem independently, record their ideas, and then reconvene and discuss and rank ideas in order of importance] ...

Of course, your choice of method for generating ideas might not only relate to the content of your task. It may be equally as important to think about some group process issues. For example, *pairs* is a particularly useful technique for generating ideas from less 'vocal' members of a group who are hesitant to call out their ideas in a brainstorming session. Similarly, *doing rounds* is a method of ensuring that all group members have the opportunity [of sharing] their ideas.

(p. 47)

Decision making

Similarly to having a range of methods for generating ideas, there are numerous methods for making group decisions. In fact, your 'generation of ideas' process will have left you with a range of options from which to choose. A decision is normally one course of action or solution that is chosen after consideration of alternative courses of action or solutions. However, sometimes groups fall into the trap of focusing on only one or two options rather than considering a range of possible options ...

Your choice of decision making method may once again be determined on either content or process issues. For example, if the group has limited time available to make the decision then *majority vote, decision by authority*, and *decision by expert* are relatively quick processes. Be aware, however, that group members may be divided into winners or losers, feel that they don't own the decision, or may disagree on the 'expert' ...

Alternatively, the decision making method your group adopts may be determined by the content of the decision. For example, your group may have generated a number of ideas regarding the topic of an oral presentation. *Group consensus*, although lengthy in process, is likely to result in a topic that all members agree on and are committed to.

(p. 49)

Conflict and problem solving in groups

Conflict in groups can sometimes prevent the group from progressing, particularly if it is not managed well. If the problems that are the cause of the conflict are not addressed, it can lead to anger, frustration or stress for individual group members and, potentially, the destruction of the group. Conflict may be caused by differences of opinion, beliefs, values, attitudes or personality. What can start as a debate or argument can escalate to threatening behaviour, direct opposition, or a stalemate. Particular skills and strategies are required to progress beyond the conflict, and to benefit from learning and positive change (Tyson, 1998). Individual differences can be a positive force for cohesion but such diversity can also be a source of conflict. Although conflict is not inevitable in all groups, it is quite common. Conflict is not always negative and may be a constructive source of change for the group.

(p. 51)

What should we do if conflict occurs?

When conflict occurs, group members face an important 'choice point'. Do we ignore the conflict, pretend it isn't there, and just try to focus on getting the task done? Or do we try to address the conflict openly, or the problems that have caused it, and risk making matters worse? Is there a risk that people will be emotionally hurt or upset further if we do, or don't, deal with the conflict? The answers to these questions, and the direction that the group heads in, depend on several factors.

One factor to consider is whether the group will be ongoing or will terminate soon, due to completion of the task. Some groups that are near completion of their task may choose not to address the conflict, as long as it doesn't prevent task completion. However, there are some distinct disadvantages of this approach. First, it may leave group members feeling unsatisfied because the unresolved conflict remains 'unfinished business'. This can continue to be a source of psychological distress for some individuals. Second, it doesn't allow the opportunity for the group to learn from working through the issues, and for individuals to learn about the impact of their behaviour on others. Many individuals benefit from this type of learning.

Another factor to consider is whether the conflict is able to be resolved. If the conflict has arisen due to a 'personality clash' between individuals, or their values and beliefs are in conflict, it is possible that the conflict cannot be entirely resolved. Nevertheless, the group members may decide to 'agree to disagree' and proceed with the task, with diminished relationship maintenance activities. Sometimes, individuals are either unwilling or unable to change their behaviour or attitudes in ways that can be tolerated by others. If the group is to continue, this will no doubt involve compromise and accommodation among the group members.

A third factor to consider is whether there is motivation to resolve the conflict among group members, particularly those who are primarily involved in the conflict. Is there a degree of goodwill on the part of each person involved?

Finally, does the group have the skills and resources necessary to facilitate problem solving, or negotiate a compromise? Would it be beneficial to involve an external facilitator or mediator? Often a mediator is viewed by group members as impartial, and that [a fair process will take place].

(pp. 51–52)

Group endings

Although there is a [considerable] amount of effort put into the early and middle stages of group development, the later stages often receive little consideration. Yet, how a group adjourns, terminates, or comes to completion can have a strong effect on an individual's attitude and behaviour in future groups.

The final stage in a group's life cycle may be either planned or spontaneous. Think about your past involvement in groups. Have some ended spontaneously? Were other endings planned? Planned dissolution usually occurs when groups have achieved their goal/s, completed their project, or have run out of time or resources. Such dissolution may occur for your group, if you formed for the purpose of working on a particular project or piece of assessment. Conversely, spontaneous dissolution is likely to result when a problem arises that makes it difficult, or impossible, for you to continue as a group. You may have experienced spontaneous dissolution in groups that were formed as support study groups – perhaps members did not contribute as agreed or failed to turn up at scheduled meeting times.

(p. 55)

Planned group endings

How much time and effort you put into your group closure may depend on the length of time you have worked together and the amount of involvement as a group. It may also depend on the extent to which you wish to learn from your group's experience so that you can enhance your effectiveness in future groups.

(p. 55)

We provide below a suggestion for how you might wish to 'end' your group's journey. This is a useful way to reflect on your group experience and plan for your future involvement in groups. Take turns with your group members to share your thoughts on one (or more) of the following (even if your group members are not interested in undertaking this activity, you can reflect on these topics yourself):

- What I learned from this group
- My most positive and most negative group experience
- What I learned from this course
- One of the skills I developed was …
- As a result of this group experience, I am now able to …
- Other things you wish to discuss.

(p. 56)

Common problems in groups

We hope that by engaging in the processes we have suggested in this chapter you will minimise problems in your group. However, we have added here a question and answer section on common problems that occur in groups.

What do we do if someone is not 'pulling their weight'?

It is important here to be certain that the way you perceive the situation reflects what is really happening. What observations of the person's behaviour can you describe? How have you interpreted these observations? Is it possible that there are alternative interpretations or explanations for the person's behaviour? Do other group members feel the same way as you about the person not pulling their weight? During formation, what did the group [agree to] in relation to workload? It may be worthwhile to review the written contract that the group developed.

If it is clear that a person is not pulling their weight, the group may need to [re-state] what their expectations are of each other and ensure that the person understands what is expected from them. This can occur in a group discussion, where each member states their progress with tasks that have been allocated to them and the anticipated completion date. It is sometimes useful to record these tasks, responsibilities and dates.

If the behaviour continues to occur, it may be necessary to address it directly with the person, stating clearly the group's concerns about an equal distribution of workload and seeking the person's ideas about how to address the concerns. This discussion can either be conducted one-to-one with the group member (by another group member), or in a group meeting. If the discussion occurs in a group meeting, the process needs careful attention to ensure that the person doesn't feel ambushed … It is important to stick to the facts and direct observations (not interpretations) of the person's behaviour, to prevent them from becoming defensive.

(p. 61)

What if someone always turns up late/leaves early?

What are the expectations, and how have those expectations [been transgressed]? What are the specific observations of the person's behaviour and what impact is it having on the group? Sometimes all that is required is for a group member to draw it to their attention ('John, I've noticed that you have been 15 minutes late for the last three meetings. This has been a bit disruptive and is affecting our progress on the task') and restate the group's expectations.

If the behaviour continues to occur, it may be necessary to address it directly with the person, stating clearly the group's concerns about arriving on time, or staying for the entire meeting, and seeking the person's ideas about how to address the concerns. This discussion can either be conducted one-to-one with the group member (by another group member), or in a group meeting. If the discussion occurs in a group meeting, the process needs careful attention to ensure that the person doesn't feel ambushed … It is important to stick to the facts and direct observations (not interpretations) of the person's behaviour, to prevent them from becoming defensive.

(p. 62)

What if I don't know what is expected of me or what my role is, or I'm unclear on the task?

Don't be afraid to ask. Often role expectations are not discussed explicitly in groups, which can lead to confusion among members. It is possible that other members are also confused about their roles.

It is necessary to be clear about the task of the group, before a discussion about roles can take place. Ensure you have read thoroughly any documentation provided to you about the task. If you are confused about the information you have, this can be a good place to start a discussion with other group members.

You may also need to seek clarification from outside the group, for example your lecturer or group facilitator, or another staff member. It is preferable to seek this clarification as early as possible, because ongoing confusion about the group's task can hinder progress.

(pp. 61–62)

What if someone always dominates the group discussion or the decision making?

This is very common in groups, and there are several ways to address it, depending on the individual involved and their willingness to listen to other group members. For example, you may need to nominate a 'gate-keeper' at each meeting. Their role is to ensure that all group members have equal 'airtime' when it comes to discussion. At times, they may need to address the dominant member directly and say, 'OK Steve, thanks for those comments ... we've heard what you have said and now we should hear what other members think'. If the dominating behaviour continues, the gatekeeper may need to escalate the intervention by saying 'Steve, it may be helpful to hear more from other members and for you to listen to what others have to say'.

If it still continues, it may be necessary to address the dominant behaviour with Steve directly 'Steve, what I have observed during the discussion is that you contribute a lot and we appreciate what you have to say. However, it is having a detrimental effect on the rest of the group. It is stopping some members from expressing their thoughts and opinions. What do you think we can do to solve this problem at future meetings?

(p. 63)

What if someone is not contributing to the discussion, or is withdrawn?

It is important to distinguish between observations and interpretations of the person's behaviour. Is it that they are not contributing at all or are they contributing to the group in a different way [from] other members? Some individuals process information differently and prefer to reflect on the discussion and state their opinion at a later time.

If the person is not contributing to any discussion and cannot be persuaded to express themselves, it may be sufficient from time to time to check with them that they are satisfied with the group's progress. If they indicate that they are, then the group can proceed. It is not productive or beneficial to attempt to force someone to express an opinion or communicate verbally if they don't want to.

(p. 64)

What if I don't like the other members of the group?

You don't have to like the people you work with, but it sometimes makes the work more enjoyable if you do. [Most people will] at sometimes in their working career have to work with people that they dislike, and it's an important skill to develop to behave professionally in these circumstances.

Have you got a clear idea about why you don't like the other member/s of the group? Is it likely to affect your contribution to the task? Is it something about their behaviour that would be easy for them to change if you were to talk to them about it, or is it something that would be very difficult for them to change? Do you feel confident that you could communicate [with them] your concerns about their behaviour in such a way that they would be not be insulted or become defensive? Is it likely to damage your working relationship with the person? These are important considerations and in some circumstances it is preferable to say nothing and be content to learn as much as possible from the experience of working with someone who is different [from] you.

(p. 64)

How do we stop ourselves from going around in circles or going 'off track'?

It can help to have an agenda for the meeting and to agree the priorities for the meeting (e.g., By the end of today's meeting we must have ...). Sometimes the discussion can get a little bit off track, or a group member can distract the group with irrelevant or trivial conversation. Appoint a process observer who is responsible for [re-focusing] the group when this happens. When the discussion begins to go down a path that is irrelevant, the process observer intervenes with a comment like 'It seems like we are getting a little off track, could we return to our discussion of ... Dean, you were saying ...'. It may also help to allow 5 minutes at the beginning or the end of the meeting for people to talk about other matters or to have a personal conversation.

(p. 65)

What happens if two people can't agree on ideas?

This can often happen, particularly if members have different backgrounds, personalities, values and attitudes. In some circumstances, group members don't have to agree on everything – different ideas and ways of thinking can be positive. Sometimes it is necessary to 'agree to disagree' on matters that are peripheral to the group's task.

However, when it comes to making a decision that will affect the group's task, a solution or a compromise is usually necessary. There are a variety of decision making processes that a group can use that can introduce some objectivity to the decision making.

(p. 65)

Conclusion

The aim of this chapter was to make working in groups easier and more fruitful for you, by suggesting several practical steps that will reduce the negative, and increase the positive, aspects of working in groups. We have taken you through some processes for forming and contracting with your group members, and planning and organising how you will work together. By following these processes, you will maximise the potential for successful outcomes from your group experience. Despite everyone's best efforts, sometimes things don't work out the way you plan, so we have also made some suggestions for overcoming difficulties you may encounter along the way.

Remember, as you work on your task, to take time to reflect on 'how' you are working together. As we said earlier in the chapter, each group experience can be reflected upon and learnt from to enhance future group experiences. And there is much to be learnt about how 'you' work in groups.

9 Final words

Improving our own learning is a high-level skill. It requires persistence, experimentation, reflection, time and effort. One of the aims of this book has been to provide ideas and strategies on ways in which we can improve how we learn. There are lots of different ways to learn and coming to understand the different ways is a first step to improving our learning. Often we need to be strategic in our choices.

Fortunately we have the opportunity to continue to improve the ways in which we learn throughout life. Many of the ideas and strategies in this book can be used outside of formal study and in our working and personal lives. Again, I wish you every success with your future studies and I hope that you find the ideas and strategies in this book to be useful.

Notes

Introduction

1   In this book, I use the term 'course' to refer to a full programme of study, i.e. a degree, certificate, diploma, etc. The term 'subject' is used to refer to the component parts of a course, which in some universities are called 'units of study' or 'modules'.

2 Study management

1   A good friend of mine is a librarian at a prestigious UK University. The tag line on her email reads 'Who says librarians aren't supposed to smell of drink' (Pym, 1955, p. 101).

3 Learning

1   The education theory that underpins this image of learning is called 'constructivism'.

2   This approach of making explicit the connections between concepts is called 'concept mapping'.

References

Ausubel, D. (1968) *Educational Psychology: A Cognitive View*, New York: Holt, Rinehart & Winston.

Big Dog, Little Dog (2008) 'Learning domains or Bloom's taxonomy'. Available at http://www.nwlink.com/~donclark/hrd/bloom.html (accessed 30 May 2008).

Bloom, B. S. (ed.) (1956) *Taxonomy of Educational Objectives: The Classification of Educational Goals*, London: Longmans, Green and Co. Ltd.

Brown, D. and Edwards, H. (eds) (2005) *Lewis's Medical–Surgical Nursing: Assessment and Management of Clinical Problems*, Sydney: Elsevier Australia.

Bruner, J. (1990) *Acts of Meaning*, Cambridge, Massachusetts: Harvard University Press.

Buzan, T. (1983) *Use your Head*, London: BBC Books.

Center for Teaching Effectiveness (2008) 'Seven Principles for good practice: enhancing student learning'. Adapted with permission from The Seven Principles Resource Center, Winona State University, Minnesota. Available at http://cte.udel.edu/TAbook/principles.html (accessed 30 May 2008).

Charles Darwin University Library (2008) 'Podcasts @ CDU Library.' Available at http://www.cdu.edu.au/library/LILL/podcasts.html (accessed 30 May 2008).

Chickering, A. W. and Gamson, Z. F. (1987) 'Seven principles for good practice in undergraduate education', *American Association for Higher Education Bulletin*, March, 3–7.

Cottrell, S. (2003) *The Study Skills Handbook*, London: Palgrave MacMillan.

Curtin University (2008) 'Startup 2008.' Available at http://startup.curtin.edu.au/study/ (accessed 30 May 2008).

Dawson, C. (2004) *Learning How to Study Again*, Oxford: howtobooks.

Ergonomics in Australia Online (2008) Available at http://www.ergonomics.com.au/ (accessed 30 May 2008).

Fowler, J., Gudmundsson, A. and Whicker, L. (2006) *Groups Work*, Queensland: Australian Academic Press.

Fraser, K. (1996) *Student Centred Teaching: The Development and Use of Conceptual Frameworks*, New South Wales: Higher Education Research Society of Australasia.

Fraser, K. (ed.) (2005) *Education Development and Leadership in Higher Education: Developing an Effective Institutional Strategy*, London: RoutledgeFalmer.

Fraser, K. and Edwards, J. (1985) 'The effects of training in concept mapping on student achievement in traditional classroom tests', *Research in Science Education*, 15: 158–165.

Gagne, E. D. (1985) *The Cognitive Psychology of School Learning*, Boston Massachusetts: Little, Brown and Co.

Georgetown University (2008) 'Avoiding plagiarism.' Available at http://ldss.georgetown.edu/acad-plagiarism.cfm (accessed 19 August 2008).

Griffith University (2008) 'Group work.' Available at http://www.griffith.edu.au/cgi-bin/frameit?http://www.griffith.edu.au/school/hsv/content/assistance/guides_skills/assistance_guides_group_work.html (accessed 30 May 2008).

HERDSA (1992) 'Challenging conceptions of teaching: Some prompts for good practice.' Sydney: Higher Education Research and Development Society of Australasia Inc.

Honey, P. and Mumford, A. (1992) *The Manual of Learning Styles*, 3rd edn, Maidenhead: P. Honey Publications.

Indiana University Writing Tutorial Services (2008) 'Plagiarism: What is it and how to recognize and avoid it.' Available at http://www.indiana.edu/~wts/pamphlets/plagiarism.shtml (accessed 30 May 2008).

Inglis, A., Ling, P. and Joosten, V. (2002) *Delivering Digitally: Managing the Transition to the Knowledge Media*, 2nd edn, London: Kogan Page.

Kolb, D. A. (1984) *Experiential Learning: Experience as the Source of Learning and Development*, New Jersey: Prentice-Hall, Inc.

Kolb, D. A. and Fry, R. (1975) 'Toward an applied theory of experiential learning', in C. Cooper (ed.) *Theories of Group Process*, London: John Wiley.

Ling, P. (2005) 'From a community of scholars to a company', in K. Fraser (ed.) *Education Development and Leadership in Higher Education: Developing an Effective Institutional Strategy*, London: RoutledgeFalmer.

Macquarie Dictionary (1991) 2nd edn, Australia: The Macquarie Library Pty Ltd.

Middlesex University (2008) 'Time management tips from students'. Available at http://www.mdx.ac.uk/www/study/Timetips.htm (accessed 30 May 2008).

Mullins, L. J. (2002) *Management and Organisational Behaviour*, 6th edn, New York: Financial Times/Prentice Hall.

Northedge, A., Thomas, J., Lane, A. and Peasgood, A. (1997) *The Sciences Good Study Guide*, Milton Keynes: Open University Press.

Novak, J. D. (1980) *Handbook for the Learning How to Learn Program*, Ithaca, New York: Cornell University Press.

Novak, J. D. (1993) 'Human constructivism: A unification of psychological and epistemological phenomena in meaning making', *International Journal of Personal Construct Psychology*, 6: 167–193.

Novak, J. D. and Gowin, D. Bob (1984) *Learning How to Learn*, Ithaca, New York: Cornell University Press.

PubMed (2008) 'Online Training.' Available at http://www.nlm.nih.gov/bsd/disted/pubmed.html (accessed 30 May 2008).

Purdue OWL (2008) 'Avoiding plagiarism.' Purdue University. Available at http://owl.english.purdue.edu/owl/resource/589/01/#resourcenav/ (accessed 30 May 2008).

Pym, B. (1955) *Less than Angels*, London: Jonathan Cape.

Ramsden, P. (2003) *Learning to Teach in Higher Education*, London: RoutledgeFalmer.

Read Write Think (2008) Available at http://www.readwritethink.org/lesson_images/lesson158/plagiarismactivity.pdf (accessed 19 August 2008).

Scholtes, P. R. (1992) *The Team Handbook*, Madison: Joiner Associates.

Sherman, L. W. (1995) 'A postmodern, constructivist and cooperative pedagogy for teaching educational psychology, assisted by computer mediated communications', in Schnase, J. L. and Cunnius, E. L. (eds) *Proceedings of CSCL '95 Conference*.

Study Guides and Strategies (2008) 'Managing time.' Available at http://www.studygs.net/timman.htm (accessed 30 May 2008).

Symington, D. and Novak, J. (1982) 'Teaching children how to learn', *Education Magazine*, 39:5, September: 13–16.

Tyson, T. (1998) *Working with Groups*, 2nd edn, South Yarra: Swinburne University of Technology.

White, R. and Gunstone, R. (1992) *Probing Understanding*, London: The Falmer Press.

Williams, J., Smithburn, J. and Peterson, J. (1980) *Lizzie Borden: A Case Book of Family and Crime in the 1890s*, Bloomington: TIS Publications Division.

Wood, J., Chapman, J., Fromholtz, M., Morrison, V., Wallace, J., Zeffane, R., Schermerhorn, J. R., Hunt, J. G. and Osborn, R. N. (2004) *Organisational Behaviour: A Global Perspective*, 3rd edn, Brisbane: John Wiley.

Index

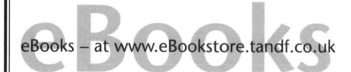
eBooks – at www.eBookstore.tandf.co.uk

A library at your fingertips!

eBooks are electronic versions of printed books. You can store them on your PC/laptop or browse them online.

They have advantages for anyone needing rapid access to a wide variety of published, copyright information.

eBooks can help your research by enabling you to bookmark chapters, annotate text and use instant searches to find specific words or phrases. Several eBook files would fit on even a small laptop or PDA.

NEW: Save money by eSubscribing: cheap, online access to any eBook for as long as you need it.

Annual subscription packages

We now offer special low-cost bulk subscriptions to packages of eBooks in certain subject areas. These are available to libraries or to individuals.

For more information please contact webmaster.ebooks@tandf.co.uk

We're continually developing the eBook concept, so keep up to date by visiting the website.

www.eBookstore.tandf.co.uk